The Online Yoga Teacher's Guide

of related interest

Developing a Yoga Home Practice
An Exploration for Yoga Teachers and Trainees
Alison Leighton with Joe Taft
ISBN 978 1 78775 704 2
eISBN 978 1 78775 705 9

Yoga Teaching Handbook
A Practical Guide for Yoga Teachers and Trainees
Edited by Sian O'Neill
ISBN 978 1 84819 355 0
eISBN 978 0 85701 313 2
Yoga Teaching Guides

THE ONLINE YOGA TEACHER'S GUIDE

Get Confident and Thrive Online

Jade Beckett

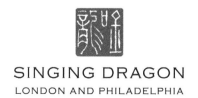

SINGING DRAGON
LONDON AND PHILADELPHIA

First published in Great Britain in 2022 by Singing Dragon
An imprint of Jessica Kingsley Publishers
An imprint of Hodder & Stoughton Ltd
An Hachette Company

1

A CIP catalogue record for this title is available from the
British Library and the Library of Congress

ISBN 978 1 83997 180 8
eISBN 978 1 83997 181 5
Premium ebook 978 1 83997 182 2

Printed and bound in Great Britain by CPI Group UK

Jessica Kingsley Publishers' policy is to use papers that are natural,
renewable and recyclable products and made from wood grown in
sustainable forests. The logging and manufacturing processes are expected
to conform to the environmental regulations of the country of origin.

Jessica Kingsley Publishers
Carmelite House
50 Victoria Embankment
London EC4Y 0DZ

www.singingdragon.com

Contents

Preface

The world of teaching yoga, Pilates and fitness classes is dramatically changing.

We came away from our traditional face to face classes to having to incorporate a range of online classes and products into our offerings, for what we thought would be a few weeks, to seeing the need to make online into a permanent part of our businesses.

Whether we like it or not, our businesses have changed forever. Students all over the world are loving the online class environments we've created – online is here to stay and is only set to boom and grow even further over the next decade.[1]

We all deserve to be able to take advantage of this. We deserve to grow our businesses, help more people and make a good amount of money while having more flexibility, without teaching more and more classes and burning ourselves out.

Maybe you...

- have been muddling through and need to up level your processes and equipment
- have been sticking your head in the sand, reluctant to start
- want to develop a membership offering
- stopped teaching and need to get teaching again
- lack confidence and feel overwhelmed trying to figure teaching online out.

The Online Yoga Teacher's Guide is here to help you with all of this.

We will cover all the essential knowledge you need to know so you can get teaching online and build a resilient business on your own terms going forwards, so even the least tech-savvy teacher can benefit.

I will help you get to the bottom of your own business, figure out what approach your students would love, put that into action and teach you the tools, show you the equipment – the how, when, where, what and why in a straightforward easy to follow way.

Ready to get confident and thriving online?

Let's do this!

A few words on *The Online Yoga Teacher's Guide*

Before we dive in to getting you thriving online, it's worth mentioning that this book is a little bit different to a lot of business books. It's specifically written by me, a yoga business owner, for you, another yoga business owner.

It isn't prescriptive or one size fits all. A lot of business books come with the masculine, corporate, willy-waving "I'm better than you" posturing and hustle culture, my way or the highway view. Which to be honest, I'm sick to the back teeth of and, frankly, makes me want to hurl. (I'm sure you feel the same!)

A yoga or wellbeing business isn't like that at all. It's holistic and we are working with people's feelings and energy, as well as our own, so we can do our jobs to our absolute best. We genuinely care about the work we do, deeply. We don't want to strong arm people, we want to support them.

Think of this more like an anti-hustle business book for businesses who want and need to work sustainably in terms of their own energy, approach and ethos.

All yoga businesses are totally different by the virtue that they are run by wonderful individuals for their own pool of students, so to say there's only one way of doing everything would be totally wrong here. Different students have different needs, quite obviously.

You might already have a pretty good idea of the sort of thing you want to do, which is amazing, or maybe you're not sure of where to even start. Which is also cool.

Each chapter is going to take you through a specific area of teaching online. We're going to start with the real foundational basics of every yoga business and then build on top of it, so we are totally clear on what we are doing for who and why, before getting into the practical hands-on elements. The idea is that we don't run before we can walk (or crawl) and go through the whole process from start to finish so you end up with the best offering/product for your students.

Each section of the book has a variety of different worksheets, videos and activities for you to complete to help you on this journey.

Copies of the worksheets and the videos are available to download from https://library.singingdragon.com/redeem using the voucher code JEWZDYR

Every single one of you who picks up this book will end up taking something totally different and have different plans and ideas based on the following chapters, and that is the beauty of this book.

My role here isn't to tell you what to do. My role is to introduce all the key considerations around each aspect of teaching online, critically discuss the options and the pros and cons of each approach and offer you a little insight into my own personal experience with my own teaching business, so you're informed and empowered to go on to make the right choice for you and you can also learn from some of my mistakes. (Yes, I do make loads of them!)

It's your business, so it is up to you to make a final call with exactly what feels right for you, and the only way to know that is for you to do the work. This is very much a case of you get out what you put in! By the end of the book you will have clarity on what you want to do, how you want to do it and be well on your way to bringing that to reality.

Think of it a little bit like having me as your pocket-sized cheerleading business coach in your pocket. You already have some, if not all, of the answers. You probably need a helping hand to get there and that's what this book is here to help you with.

Onwards!

Intentions

We're going to kick off with a short journaling activity to help frame our aims and what we want to get out of working through this book.

Journaling is a wonderful practice that you might be familiar with and use in conjunction with your yoga practice, or maybe you've never tried it. Journaling is primarily a tool for exploration. A safe space to explore who you are, what you feel and your thoughts by jotting whatever comes to mind down on paper. This gives you time and space to reflect and revisit whatever you've written over days, weeks, months and years. You can journal freely and write as much or as little as you want, or you can use prompts, or a prompted exercise like this one we're going to start with.

It essentially allows us to get everything out of our heads (literally) and make everything a little quieter. In this case we're going to use what comes out of this journaling session to help keep you on track and give you a focus to the work you do and allow you to explore those areas thoroughly.

Journaling Exercise: Intention Setting

Equipment needed: timer, notebook and a pen

- Sit down with your notebook and pen.
- Set a timer for 10–15 minutes.
- Spend a few moments journaling around each of these prompts:
  - Why did I pick up this book?
  - What are the three things I need help with the most?
  - What questions on teaching online do I need help finding answers for?
  - How do I feel about teaching online right now?
  - How do I want to feel about teaching online after I've completed this book?

As you read and work through each chapter, I also encourage you to journal during the process. Write a few words about how you feel, anything that comes up, any realisations you have. This will be helpful for you to refer back to as you work through the later chapters and will help with our final exercise at the end of the book.

Video 1: Visualisation Exercise can be downloaded from https://library.singingdragon.com/redeem using the voucher code JEWZDYR

Your why

There is a reason why you are a yoga teacher. One of the things most teachers say is "I love helping people" which is, of course, wonderful, but it's not a unique thing to you. In reality, it is much deeper than that and more personal too for most of us.

It's something that is hard to explain to another person, especially someone outside our industry. It might be a series of experiences, a wish for a simpler life, freedom or something you can't quite put your finger on. There's a magic and something almost ancient about that why, a knowing in your bones, a deeper connection or calling.

Before we get into the faux-meaty stuff around the topic at hand, you need to connect with your why. Teaching isn't easy, we all know that. Learning to teach online, researching your Ideal Student, getting all the tech, systems and everything else in place is a serious undertaking. It'll be hard. It'll annoy you. You will get frustrated, and you might want to give up. All that is okay. It's so normal and we will get through it together, I promise! And one thing that will help you is having a visual reference in your workspace that is a representation of your *why*. When things get hard, you can quickly refocus and reconnect.

We're going to spend a bit of time making a vision board. If you aren't familiar, this is essentially a moodboard or visual reference highlighting everything that reminds you of your why. It could be an old-skool paper board that you cut and stick your images on to (*such fun!*) or it could be a digital one that you set as your laptop and phone background.

Whichever version you choose the principles are the same – once you're happy with it, have it somewhere you can see it consistently: your office space, the space you teach in or wherever else. You want to spend a couple of minutes each day or whenever you are working through this book looking at it to allow that connection with your why to flourish and grow stronger.

Vision Boarding
Equipment needed:

Paper vision board: paper, magazines, Pinterest, scissors, glue and a printer

or

Digital vision board: PowerPoint/Canva, Pinterest

and a spare couple of hours

- Sit down with a blank sheet of paper and a pen.
  - Write the word *"why"* in the middle.
  - Set a timer for 10 minutes – if you finish earlier, that's fine.
  - Jot down all the words and phrases that leap to mind immediately.
  - Be guided by your intuition and try not to force it.
- Sit down with a tea/coffee/drink of choice and browse the internet or magazines for images for your board.
  - Anything that calls to you, even if it makes *no sense* right now – select it for inclusion on your board.
  - The number you need will depend on the size of your board.
  - Have a mix of images and quotes.
    » Quotes could be single words that resonate, longer phrases or sayings from well-known people, or reminders you know you need.
    » You might want to include affirmations: "I am a great yoga teacher and business owner" or headline goals: "a thriving yoga membership".
- Arrange all your images, quotes and any other visual references onto your physical or digital vision boards.
- Once you're happy, display it somewhere you can see it throughout your day.
- If you've gone digital, set it as your laptop background and resize to your phone too.

Now we've got ourselves clear on what our intentions are and what that why is, let's talk about why teaching online is such a great idea.

Chapter 1

WHY ONLINE?

Online is a very different approach to our traditional business model and way of working, and that change can seem really intimidating at first glance with so many things to think about.

Feeling overwhelmed, not sure where to start, the worry of finding students and all those not so nice feelings are a natural reaction to making such a fundamental change. This emerging online world is something so far outside the comfort zone of many yoga teachers. It's okay to feel like this right now, and you aren't alone.

The great news is, teaching online doesn't need to make you feel like this. Teaching online provides us with a whole host of opportunities that haven't been available to previous generations of teachers. It's a whole new way of working and that is a hugely exciting thing! Change is great and it'll bring great things for all of us if we embrace the challenge, welcome it in and see where it takes us.

We are at a once in a generation point in our profession where we can make a big change for the better. These changes are going to benefit our students and mean we can help more people, while making what we do work better for us too. It's a winner all round.

In this chapter we're going to discuss a few of the many reasons to incorporate an online offering into your yoga business on an ongoing, long term basis.

Protecting your livelihood by diversifying your income

As yoga teachers we traditionally rely solely on in-person classes of our own, for studios, 1:1s or corporate clients with a client base limited to our local areas.

We provide a service (a class) and get paid for the service each time we deliver it. This is known as active revenue, meaning we can only earn the money for that particular class once and it requires our active participation for that to happen. The money we make is very rarely recurring. People pay each week or every few weeks and that means we must be actively on top of reminding people to book into class, chasing payments and admin.

Burnout is a big issue for yoga teachers. We've spent years running around our towns and cities teaching four or five classes a day, every day just to scrape by, barely making ends meet and being scared of falling ill or taking much needed time off. If you are a teacher who works in studios, you might be under pressure to promote the studio's classes under threat of being dropped if the numbers in classes drop. None of this is sustainable energetically – or a great way to live either.

Yoga teachers are exploited heavily and taken advantage of by many yoga studios. Yoga studios paying ethically and offering employee status are few and far between and stories of exploitation are rampant; most yoga teachers have at least one of these stories in their circles of teacher friends. We're treated as gig economy workers, paid a very low wage for the work done, have no sick pay, holiday pay or employment rights, and can be dropped without notice or recourse. We're at a period of change in the yoga world with Yoga Unions in the US and in the UK who are actively campaigning for this situation to change.

Until that change happens, we are left in an incredibly precarious situation because, as a business model, it is unbelievably vulnerable to external influences beyond our immediate control. If we take a holiday or get hurt we don't get paid because we can't carry out the service if we aren't physically present. If our venues choose or are forced to close, we lose that income altogether.

Love and light isn't a globally accepted currency (as much as many yoga teachers would love it to be!). We need to be able to make a good consistent level of income to pay our bills, have a pension for when we are older and continue to do our jobs in a way that doesn't burn us out or is totally at odds with the underpinning philosophical teachings of yoga.

At the end of the day, how can we teach principles like ahimsa to our students in classes if we allow ourselves to be treated poorly and don't look after ourselves in our wider work? I know this is a challenging point to raise. I'd love you to take a few minutes to process this by exploring this point and the journaling exercise below.

Journaling Exercise: Current Work and Me

Equipment needed: timer, notebook and a pen

- Sit down with your notebook and pen.
- Set a timer for 10–15 minutes.
- Spend a few moments journaling around each of these prompts:
  - Does my current working situation allow me to be comfortable financially? Answer Yes or No, then elaborate on this point.
  - Am I looking after myself with my work commitments?
  - How am I treated by the studios I work for?
  - Am I happy being treated this way?
  - If money wasn't an issue, would I choose to work there?

There is a better way. If we can develop our own offerings, we can do less of this precarious work. We can say no to work that makes us feel rubbish. We can be selective about where and how we choose to teach because we are creating our own sources of income and taking charge of what we do, with unlimited earning potential and not solely relying on studios for all our work.

We are protecting ourselves and saying a hard no to poor treatment to boot. Whether you're on holiday, get hurt or something else happens – you've got something to fall back on and won't lose all your income entirely. It effectively spreads the risk so if something happens in one area (for example, if you can't teach in-person classes) your online offering is still there to work for you.

Teaching online offers us one way to do this. It offers us the opportunity to create a passive income as well as another active stream of revenue. It also allows us to create recurring revenue into our businesses where we get paid continuously for an existing product. This is known as diversifying our income, simply meaning that we have multiple ways to bring money into our businesses and protect ourselves.

Teaching online falls into two strands: on demand classes and live classes (these could be interactive, or one way streamed – more on this later).

On demand classes fall into the passive income category. We do the work once by filming and creating a single class, then that class exists and continues to earn us money either via a membership offering, bundles or individual classes on a lifetime access purchase or rental basis. This income can come in on a recurring basis automatically, so we don't even have to do anything.

Live online classes are another active source of revenue as we can teach these from anywhere that has a good internet connection either on an occasional basis or as a part of our ongoing offerings.

Reach

Usually when we teach a class the people who are in the class live fairly local to the studio, hall or gym we are teaching in. There's a finite number of people in the area who want to take yoga classes, who can make a class on a particular day and time and who don't already practise with another teacher in your area.

The internet is immune to geographical or time zone constraints and significantly broadens the number of people who we can reach with our classes.

We have an opportunity to reconnect with students who have moved away, even people in other countries, and that is an amazing thing that is brand new to our generation of yoga teachers.

Convenience

Going to a yoga class usually looks something like this: get dressed, leave home or work on time, get in car and drive to studio/class, find somewhere to park, pay for parking, make sure to arrive early enough to settle in and get a great spot, do the class then reverse the process to go back home. That is hugely time consuming and a big chunk out of any student's day.

Online classes are so much more convenient to fit yoga into day-to-day life. The process is significantly less stressful as it's as simple as picking a video and hitting play when you are ready or clicking a link with a couple of minutes to go before the class starts.

Online classes cut the time requirement down significantly, the time it takes to do the class is the length of the class plus a couple of min-utes to roll out a mat and put it away again. It saves a lot of hassle for time-stretched people. Many students who come to yoga are profession-als, parents, have generally busy lives so anything that is convenient and makes their lives easier is highly valued.

In my experience, once students have tried online offerings and have realised the convenience online classes offers them, there's a desire to retain access as well as having the option to go to a few in-person classes too. The students you have often end up spending more on their yoga and doing live classes as well as on demand ones and getting even more value from their practice, which is a huge win for them because they feel great and a win for you financially too.

Future proofing

The growth of online fitness classes and wellbeing platforms is accelerat-ing driven by consumer interest in healthy lifestyles, lack of time and the demand surge caused by COVID-19, with an expectation for this market to be worth $59.23 billion by 2027.[2]

This creates an opportunity for each yoga teacher and their own unique business. By getting in on this opportunity early, we have the chance to grow rapidly along with this change in behaviour and have access to our Ideal Students all over the world, and the chance to grab a piece of a much larger market.

Objections: the experience and tech smarts

It's important to note that the experience online isn't identical to an in-person class. This is the most common objection that students tend to voice when I've surveyed my own classes. They are reluctant to change, don't like it and see different as not as good. The second most common objection is people feeling they just aren't tech savvy and thinking it'll be too difficult for them to participate.

The ones who've decided to give it a go absolutely love online classes and think they're brilliant. You're always going to have objections or things come up for some people, others won't even blink and be up for it without a second thought.

Of course, online is a different experience. We're not in the same space sharing the same energy, the giggles, the longer pre and post-class chats while we're online. That doesn't mean that it's a poor substitute, it just means we need to be creative with how we create community and offer those little extra special things to create an experience for our students and communicate that different can be a great thing. We'll dive into this in more detail later on.

The good news is there are lots of options for making class easy for less tech-savvy students too, from selecting easier to use software to prioritising the simplicity of that student's journey. Again, we will cover this in detail in later chapters.

There will always be students and teachers who love going to an in-person class either occasionally or on a really regular basis, and there will always be students who love online now they've tried it. There will also be students who just don't click with the online world, and that is okay too. It's up to you to design an offering to suit and focus your energy on attracting the people it is suited towards.

As teachers, online offers us the opportunity to create a business model offering a selection of classes in different formats to suit the widest range of people possible, allowing us to build and scale our businesses sustainably.

Chapter 2

BUSINESS OWNER LIFE

Mindsets, Mental Health, Money and Confidence

"I'm not a good enough yoga teacher."
"I need to charge less to attract people."
"It's a hobby so I can do it really cheap."
"I should put full-length classes on my YouTube channel."
"Everyone else is offering Pay What You Can... I should do this too."

Does this sound like you? Yes?

Well, this is the chapter where we're going to dive into some of the common thoughts, feelings and experiences every single business owner has at some point or another.

There's a huge misconception out there that business is easy. I don't think anything I say here would prepare you for how tough it can be; it must be experienced. The idea pushed out into the world is that it's easy to be successful, no mindset issues ever come up, it's always sunshine and rainbows. Actually, it's really important that we are transparent and authentic and say openly, yes, these things happen. It helps all yoga teachers feel less alone, knowing there are others who feel exactly the same way. It's also important to note that running a business isn't for everyone, which is also totally okay.

These beliefs and mindsets infiltrate your business and prevent you from making decisions, taking action and building the successful online yoga business of your dreams. They can also drive you to taking actions that aren't aligned, are disrespectful or ill advised. If you know it could come up, that knowledge is even more helpful and gives you the opportunity to get to grips with it and nip it in the bud before it turns into a major problem. Only when we understand these issues, how they manifest for each of us individually, can we start to move past these and get on with the job of researching then building our online offerings.

I know this section is possibly the most confronting in this book. It may well bring up some feelings for you. You might want to say "Jade, what a load of rubbish!" It might feel like I'm staring deep into your soul. That's fine! I am sorry for any not so nice emotional responses this chapter brings up for you.

Please know that everything said here is from a place of love and nurturing. My job here is to help you make great decisions and build something sustainable for yourself that also uplifts our whole profession, and to do that I'm going to have to share some hard truths! I wouldn't be doing you or this project justice if I shove this under the carpet and glossed over this stuff purely because it's hard to hear.

There are a lot of deep-seated elements to learn about in this chapter and this is a top-level overview of the common mindset, confidence and business acumen things that come up with the yoga teachers I work with every day and some I've worked through myself.

I'd suggest taking some time to read this section and digest it, and maybe revisit the points you feel are very relevant to you. You might want to do a few short reflective journaling practices to help you process and understand the concepts we talk about, and how they show up in your business. I won't prompt these here, because each reader's experience will be different. If you feel any strong emotions, that is definitely a point to revisit in your journal.

Let's dive in!

Scarcity mindset and limiting beliefs: examples and tactics

Scarcity mentality refers to people seeing life as a finite pie, so that if one person takes a big piece, that leaves less for everyone else.[3]

Being in a scarcity mindset is often a result of limiting beliefs and both of these are hugely common things that every business owner experiences and struggles with, especially at times of growth, pivot or stepping into the unknown in their business.

This mindset is an energetically draining space to be in. It takes up a lot of energy to be worrying about what others are doing, why they have teaching slots for XYZ Studio and you don't, why their classes are busy, how they got so many clients with seemingly no effort. Even writing that was exhausting! It's not a nice place to be.

Scarcity mindset takes you away from where you should be directing your energy – on yourself, your success and not worrying about what *"Bendy Wendy 10,000 HR YTT in the Lulu pants"* is doing.

It can also make you take desperate action, doing things like actively setting out to solicit students away from other teachers by commenting on their posts, dropping your prices to below cost or running classes at a loss. None of these are good things to do ethically or respectfully of other yoga teachers or yourself either. It really is like cutting your nose off to spite your face.

Limiting beliefs originate in our subconscious mind. The subconscious mind is the deeper layer underneath the daily chatter and thoughts we have in our conscious mind.

The limiting beliefs are the stories we've heard from being small, the things we've been told by parents, society and conditioned to believe are true. These are the things we "should" do – go to university, get a corporate job, hustle culture, £10k months as a success measure.

Here's the kicker though…none of these things are true. It's our subconscious telling us things to railroad us. It's that little devil sitting on our shoulder talking negatively. This makes it really challenging to identify and spot.

Limiting beliefs like to sabotage our potential for success by trying to get us to act and work in line with those beliefs. When we are doing things that are outside our comfort zone or outside of what society deems as the norm, this is when they crop up and try to get us back in our boxes.

Teaching yoga is a profession that is outside of these societal norms by its very nature. It's hugely unsociable (when we're told that working 9–5 is the only way to be successful), it can be quite spiritual and is always person centred, which isn't understood and isn't a huge part of our western culture.

When we step outside of these societal norms we get pushback from ourselves at a deeper subconscious level and from others at an overt level as well. We are going against the grain and what society deems to be a usual route and the accepted way of working or success.

Given all this conditioning we see day in day out across our societies – not only limited to the work we do, but gender roles, being a woman doing the unexpected, running a business that isn't rooted in hustle culture – it is no wonder we are fighting ourselves and others to bring our visions into reality. It isn't your fault.

Here's a couple of examples that crop up regularly in the yoga community:

"I'm not good enough."

Maybe you had a school teacher who said you could try harder even when you were trying your best. Now you get this horrible impostor type feeling and always feel people are going to think you're a fraud.

"What if I fail/no one signs up/I look silly?"

Maybe you had parents who pushed you academically and you felt you might get punished if you didn't get top grades. This changes into over-perfectionism as an adult. Now you stress if you mess up, something isn't exactly how you want it, you don't sell out your classes. You might experience high functioning anxiety and that manifests through over-working, the inability to make important decisions.

All of these examples, societal conditioning and beliefs can cause real issues within your yoga business. The great news: any limiting belief can be tackled and undone with some strategies, and support from a therapist or business coach (depending on the circumstance) if you feel it would be beneficial.

How do we deal with this? We need to do the work internally. Learning about these things that come up, educating those external people where we can that what we do is valuable and valid work and learning not to listen to the haters. Not everyone will want to listen. It will trigger people. That's fine and entirely on them, not you. It's about each yoga teacher out there believing in what we do with full confidence.

Ultimately, "I'm not good enough" comes from the worry that there isn't a place for you as a yoga teacher and it leads to decisions that don't benefit your business or yoga teaching as a profession.

This belief that there isn't a place for you couldn't be further from the truth. There is space for us all. Really, there is.

If ten yoga teachers taught the exact same class, you'd end up with ten totally different experiences in terms of energy, feel, direction. Why?

Because each of those ten teachers is an individual drawing from their unique experiences and learnings. Their individuality and authenticity are what is creating the class experience and magic for each of those students.

You are the only one who can do you.

There is a place for you as a teacher and your offerings.

Your students choose to come to your class because you resonate with them. Not because you're the cheapest or anything else. They love your style, flair and experiences in class and that cannot be replicated by anyone else.

Perfectionism

Perfectionism is a funny one, because it is lauded, valued and idolised in the corporate world and in our societies generally.

In experience, though, perfectionist tendencies are a mask for high functioning anxiety. Perfectionism is a real enemy as it causes massive indecision, worry and spending hours endlessly doing jobs that should take a few minutes because *it has to be perfect* always.

You're not 100 per cent happy with the thing you've been working on, so you don't launch it? You won't let anyone else to do the job for you because it won't be how you want it? Yep! Ever spent 2 hours writing a single email? I know I have.

There's an approach I will introduce you to that is absolutely revolutionary for perfectionists: The Good Enough Approach.

It is a tried and tested approach that was introduced me to some time ago that I use myself every single day to wage war against my perfectionism and it has been super helpful, so I thought I would share it with you too.

The Good Enough Approach is a method you can use to identify if the thing you're obsessing on or spending too much time doing is going to make a difference or an impact (therefore needs a lot of attention) or is something that is or can be Good Enough to do the job.

Worksheet 2.1 is The Good Enough Approach Checklist. You can use this as a checklist, a worksheet or as a flowchart and apply it to anything you are trying to do and there is a copy of this to help you here. It is designed to help you nail down what you actually need to do within your business and make those items fit for purpose.

When we are creating in our business, you'll find that each of the tasks we need to do regularly fall into one of the following categories: functional, promotional and operational.

The functional items in your business are the things you use to capture information and record data. They're not fancy or design-led, they are a means to an end.

Promotional items are the things you use to promote your business, like your social media posts across all your channels, any worksheets or documents that students will receive, your videos, website and so on. They're the things students will see, interact with and touch as they engage with your business. These sometimes need to be functional by communicating key information like dates, times and costs, for example, but also on brand and look smart too.

Operational items are the systems that keep the cogs whirring away in your business, like payment processing, invoices, your booking system; the bits that make your business work. These are often not things students interact with on a deeper basis beyond the surface level of how they look. These can also be functional in that they are a means to an end for you as well as the student.

Some examples are:

- A booking agreement for a 1:1 client: It doesn't need to be pretty; it needs the right words on it. That's Good Enough. Don't faff about making it super pretty and designed. It's a functional document that communicates the agreement between you and your client.
- Your website: You might want a pretty welcome slideshow full of images showing what you do. But that won't sell memberships or classes. A single image and an About Me page is Good Enough. This is something that is promotional, operational and functional.
- Booking system: Can students buy a class from you, is it easy to use and for people to pay? Yes? That's Good Enough. This is an example of an operational and functional task.

It will make your teeth itch as a recovering perfectionist, but it will change your life.

THE GOOD ENOUGH APPROACH CHECKLIST

What is the objective?	
Is it? (tick all that apply)	☐ Functional – for recording information ☐ Promotional – flyers, graphics, for selling or needs branding ☐ Operational – processes for students to use or access services
What information/ processes need to happen to fulfil the objective? e.g. a booking agreement needs terms and conditions (T&Cs) in an easy to read way with minimal branding	**LIST OF ESSENTIALS** ☐ ☐ ☐ ☐ ☐ ☐ ☐ ☐ ☐ ☐ ☐ ☐ ☐ ☐ ☐ ☐ ☐ ☐
Does your item have all the essential info present?	☐ **YES** (continue!) ☐ **NO** (check checklist)
Does it need full branding applying? e.g. promotional/ operational items that are student facing Done?	☐ **YES** (add it!) ☐ **NO** ↓ (GOOD ENOUGH) ☐ **YES** ↓ (GOOD ENOUGH)

Money

Money is a controversial topic in the yoga industry and is worthy of a section in its own right due to the scale of the issues around money and how this can really hold us back from making the income we deserve from our businesses.

Talking about money in the yoga world pretty much always leads to arguments and objections, sometimes because of lack of appreciation of the wider issues and dynamics at play, limiting beliefs or just not wanting to listen. That's okay as well; not everyone is ready to have this conversation and see what we are doing as what it is – a business and industry worth billions globally.

Money is seen by some as being dirty and at odds with the roots of yoga because back when yoga was first shared, money never changed hands. There was however, an "exchange". An exchange of bed and board, clothing or something else for the class the guru taught.

Charging for a class is no different. It is an exchange of money for your time, creativity and energy that is put into each and every class you teach.

We live in a capitalist society where money is a requirement for everything we need to live – food, water, shelter, electricity and heat as well as being able to cover the costs of running a yoga business at a bare minimum. Like I said earlier, love and light isn't an acceptable method of currency. So, we must charge fair and appropriate rates and not settle for less.

So why do we insist on giving so much away for free or so little?

It comes down to a mixture of simply not knowing or using any business acumen to research the market, limiting beliefs and scarcity mindset, plus lack of confidence around knowing and charging your worth via fairly set and ethical fees:

- the lens – seeing yoga teaching as a hobby, not a business – *"I don't need to profit from it because it's for fun"*
- the perpetuating belief in society that being a yoga teacher isn't a valid choice (It is!)
- gender and pay equality – societal lag of pay and value between men and women
- scarcity mindset

  - mindset challenges around charging your worth
  - freelance pay and exploitation
- confidence.

The lens: yoga as a hobby

Let's get away from this idea of teaching yoga as a hobby, and it being acceptable to make no money from it.

If you teach yoga, you run a business. Even if it is one class per week. Even if you have another job. You own a beautiful, small business. Businesses must break even as a minimum, not run at a loss.

You might love it like a hobby; most teachers love what they do and feel hugely passionate about it. However, the hobby only/no profit mindset is really limiting to yourself and other yoga teachers everywhere, particularly those who need to make a living from teaching yoga as their sole source of income.

Tough love incoming… If you offer classes for a tiny fee or totally free online when you have another job (because it's a hobby/fun, therefore it doesn't matter to you financially what you make) what message does that send out to consumers of yoga? Spend a few moments reflecting on this, and either think about it or jot down some words in your journal.

It really sends out the message that what we do as yoga teachers isn't valuable, which couldn't be further from the truth. When you lowball and undervalue yourself, you are contributing to the problem and making it even harder for any yoga teachers to be paid fairly and earn a decent living, regardless of whether they teach part time or full time.

Low fees breed more low fees and when you decide you need more income you lose your classes because someone else is following in your footsteps, treating it like a hobby and thinks it's okay to teach that class for the equivalent of less than the minimum wage. When you set or accept low fees you make fair market-informed fees look extortionate when they aren't in reality. The other thing you might not appreciate is you could well be taking income away from another teacher and leaving them struggling. It changes yoga into a commodity like loo roll. There's no artistry or skill, it's something that has very little value, and no one can afford to be a yoga teacher any more. Please. Stop. Doing. This.

I know absolutely, hand on heart, this outcome isn't the intention here. However, look at the optics from the perspective of a student. You might be doing it because you can and you want to be nice, but those students certainly are not thinking that. They're developing a mindset along the lines of "yoga should be free; it is a basic right to have access to yoga – I do not ever want to pay for my yoga". And where does that leave us? Up the proverbial creek without a paddle because we've made our work have no value.

This hobbyist approach provides fuel for poor treatment, the commoditisation of yoga, the devaluation of the work we do and it's a spiral we need to be aware of.

There's sometimes a resistance around acknowledging ourselves as business people because of the energy around business culture and feeling a disconnect with that. I know this is something I don't connect with, and never have. As I mentioned at the start of the this, corporate business can sometimes feel very hustle, financially driven and masculine and doesn't resonate or feel authentic to ourselves within a profession that is at its heart driven by connection with others and service. It's okay to not resonate with this corporate business approach.

As yoga teachers, a lot of us have a goal of helping others and the idea of *how can I help as many people as possible* is a wonderful way of working out what feels authentic to you and helping you move into a more strategic, business-led way of working without the icky feeling.

Once you've got there and have an understanding of what you need to charge to make a viable living, a lot of these low pay issues just aren't an issue any more. You say a hard no to crap pay and negotiate better terms like a liveable basic fee and a bonus on top per head over a minimum number. You know how to set a fair fee for your own classes and online memberships, too (more on this later). You're confident in your rates, you know why they are set like that. You can even share what your fees cover with your students if you want a shiny gold star for ethical conduct and transparency.

I think this does a huge service for students too. They can see exactly what they are paying for and understand in depth why our rates are as they are and appreciate the incredible value they receive. As yoga teachers and educators, part of our job is to clue our students in on these struggles. It's authentic; it allows students to be critical of where they choose to spend their money. We don't have to pretend everything is hunky dory in yoga land, when that is far from the truth.

Yoga as a profession

Teaching yoga is a valid profession that is also hugely commercially viable. The yoga industry is worth over £900 million in the UK alone.[4] Interest in yoga is growing significantly, with 460,000 UK participants each week and the industry growing by 6 per cent annually.[5] In any book, that is a huge business and yoga teachers are essential to this. Trains can't run without train drivers. Yoga classes can't happen without teachers to teach them.

So why are we having the issue of not being paid like the professionals we are? It's an interesting conundrum with lots of facets and factors.

Gender and pay equality

The yoga industry is heavily dominated by women[6] and, as a society, we are currently 135 years[7] away from achieving pay equality between men and women – truly shocking to write in 2021.

In the yoga industry we have a predominant workforce who have been subject to systemic inequality throughout their working lives – being paid less purely because of their gender. All of this leads to more mindset issues around money, the prices being charged and the value of the work we do.

It is seen as socially acceptable for a man to ask for a raise or name a rate of pay, but if a woman does this it is seen as overly ambitious, too much. This societal attitude and inequality is a huge problem that appears as a limiting belief in our businesses. It's no wonder we worry endlessly about being seen as professional business owners, don't take what we do seriously and don't charge the rates we deserve. We grow up seeing hustle culture males being lauded as the model of success on TV and in the media. We rarely see a woman from an industry like ours up there challenging that status quo.

This is recognised at a governmental level with various departments in governments across the globe set up to address fair pay.

It is important for women to be aware of this issue and ensure we are paid fairly. Women need to have an equal seat at the table and when we work for ourselves it is down to us to do the work for the good of yoga teachers everywhere. We deserve to work and ensure that we charge fair prices in line with the market rate. Money isn't dirty.

If you'd like to learn some more about the Gender Pay Gap, Close the Gap is a wonderful organisation that researches and campaigns on this issue and has lots of resources on this topic.

Repeat after me:

I am worthy of making an income from yoga.
I own a yoga business.
My business deserves success.

Mindset challenges around money and charging your worth

Many yoga teachers do not charge their worth for one or a combination of reasons relating to limiting beliefs, scarcity mindsets or from not knowing about the need to do research to set pricing.

Classes are frequently offered at well below market rate (as low as £3 in the UK for a 60-minute online class). We need to shift the needle, research and charge our worth, as we discussed earlier in this chapter. We need to protect our income by monetising full-length classes and not giving this product away for free.

Pay what you can is commonly offered, with good intentions (as kindhearted yoga teachers). The problem is that this results in so many teachers teaching classes for below minimum wage. It's open to abuse because people sometimes take advantage of this kindness rather than allowing it to be used as intended.

When we shift our mindset to that of a business owner, wonderful things happen.

- We are charging a rate that uplifts the whole profession, ensuring more of us are paid fairly. It helps everyone.
- We don't give away products we can monetise for free, creating demand and more business for our paid offerings.
- We attract great students who are invested in their growth as yoga students who keep coming back, rather than wasting energy attracting people who are just there for the freebies and who don't want to pay us.

Freelance pay and exploitation

It would be remiss to write about money and not talk about the sad fact that teachers are often subject to labour exploitation in the yoga world: working for below the living wage,[8] in poor conditions without sick or holiday pay, and having no protection if the studio decides to cancel or cut back our classes, sometimes without notice.

We are, in effect, gig economy workers when we provide our services to studios. It leaves us vulnerable and unable to negotiate better terms. After all, the studio could give that slot to someone else prepared to accept those terms. Teaching slots are in demand and the volume of teachers being churned out means there is always someone else waiting in the wings to take any timetable slots.

Yoga teachers then feel pressured into settling for something that is far lower than our value, while studios get away with this sub-par treatment as there is no accountability.

The "karma yogi" or "dharma" argument is sometimes used to justify additional unpaid labour like cleaning bathrooms, mats and studios, working reception and dealing with student enquiries. This is often thrown in as a flat fee to do this additional work as well as teach the class, meaning the real pay for that class is incredibly low and in some cases below minimum wage.

This perpetuates the habitual scarcity mindset that teachers often experience. We feel expendable and feel we need to be grateful for these opportunities that sometimes take advantage of us. This leads to chronic undervaluing and commoditisation of our skills, as we don't value our work because we're only ever told we're worth a small fee.

If we create our own revenue streams and our own offerings, we can start to change the tide and stand up for our profession because we're in effect creating our own online studios in direct competition. We won't need to solely rely on studio classes for our income and will be empowered to say no to situations that aren't beneficial.

If you are in the UK or the US, we are fortunate to be at the forefront of the Yoga Teacher's Unionisation movement, which is actively creating yoga in action to change some of these issues.

Let's be the change we want to see.

Other ways scarcity and limiting beliefs can manifest in your business

Scarcity manifests in lots of different ways and each person's experience will differ slightly.

The common thread is that many of these are self-sabotaging, negative self-talk related and are not nice things to experience. They might be coupled with stress and anxiety symptoms or other externally noticeable factors.

Some examples are:

- undervaluing and undercharging for your classes
- saying yes to things you want to say no to
- falling into a scroll hole: spending hours looking at other yoga teachers' content and presence on social media, comparing yourself to them
- the feeling you aren't good enough
- rushing into creating classes that don't align with your ethos
- getting scared and giving up on planned launches last minute
- popping your full-length classes on YouTube for free, sabotaging your on demand offering in the process.

The way scarcity mindset and limiting beliefs shows up for each person is totally individual and it is worth getting to know what this looks like for you. Spend some time jotting your own experiences and thoughts down on Worksheet 2.2.

MY MINDSET

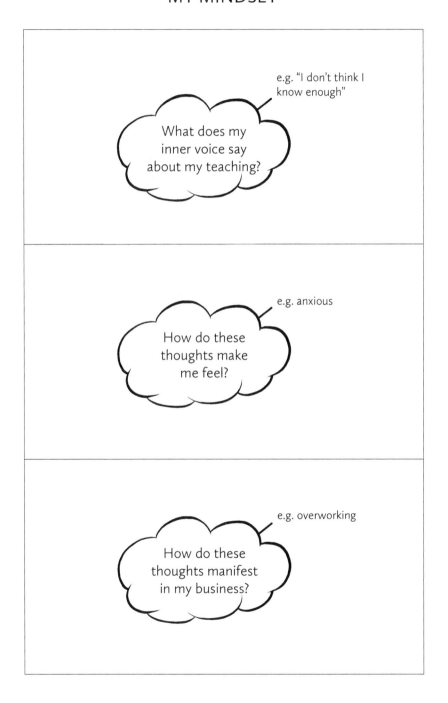

Confidence

There are a few factors for building your confidence as a business owner:

- your plan: spending time researching, getting to know your Ideal Students and developing a plan to attract them (we will talk about this in the coming chapters)
- knowing your limiting beliefs and working to undo them
- recognising how your scarcity mindset appears
- building confidence in your abilities and knowledge
- leaning into your authenticity.

When you are being authentic to your business and yourself, you're coming from a place of abundance and leading with *how can I serve/help* rather than *what can I get*.

This is instantly a more positive approach for your business because you know at a deep level who you are as a teacher, you are able to look for opportunities more easily and make decisions with confidence because you know where you want to be, and have a clear plan how to get there.

Welcome the fear

Remember teaching that first ever yoga class and being scared?

That fear is a totally natural reaction to being a beginner at anything. The first time we do or try any new thing, be it setting up a business, teaching yoga, learning to drive or anything else, it will happen.

It is a primal reaction to something unknown, and the firing of our sympathetic nervous system. We literally cannot help it – our brain sees the activity as threatening. The amygdala analyses the threat, the hypothalamus activates the sympathetic nervous system and gets us primed and ready to get up and run for the hills. Our brain doesn't care we're trying to teach a yoga class; it thinks we potentially need to run from a bear! Sweaty palms, racing heart and spiking cortisol and adrenaline into our systems.[9]

This is when those limiting beliefs can kick in hard and try to keep you small and stop you doing the things you want to – telling you to stay small, get a corporate job like you're supposed to; the perfectionism kicks in hard and says the product isn't good enough.

The first step? Knowing that what you're doing is a scary thing and that it takes courage to do it. Then do it anyway.

Any action, even if it is a little messy (PS no one else will think this, it's your Inner Perfectionist trying to sabotage you), takes you on the journey to where you want to go. If you don't do anything, nothing happens or changes.

Running a business on your own is a very scary thing. There's no one to bounce your ideas off, no one to hold you accountable (or tell you off for watching Netflix when you should be building your website).

If we want to get anywhere, we've got to go through the fear by feeling it and doing the thing instead of letting us talk ourselves out of success. This ultimately makes the activity less threatening, so we feel more comfortable next time, as well as building our confidence and skill. We've literally got to feel that fear.

Who are your cheerleaders?

The yoga industry is very solitary by design. We are very often on our own all day aside from the classes we teach. The classes we teach are often at really unsociable times early in the morning, in the evening or on weekends and when we are off our friends and families are at work, and vice versa, and that is really lonely and very challenging to adjust to. Many of us got into teaching because we enjoy being around and helping people and this just isn't talked about enough.

As I mentioned in the previous section, there's also very little accountability because it is literally you and yourself in your business, especially in the early days when you really need support and encouragement whilst you are finding your feet.

It is a great idea to develop a circle of yoga or fitness teachers around you. This could be something more informal like having a group chat with friends you've made on teacher trainings, some teachers in your local area or a virtual group on Facebook or via a paid coaching/forum membership.

You could also explore a slightly more formal arrangement like an Accountability Buddy. This could be someone who you pair up with; you agree to regular calls and catch ups and help each other through your struggles.

Hiring a business coach who has done what you want to do is also another excellent way to work. This is great because you have someone there who can give you sound advice as well as holding you accountable and help you to get systems and processes in place, so you get confident with what you are doing.

Most of the time you have a pretty good idea of what the answers are on an intuitive level. You might feel like you need a hand or a little support to get over the line, confirm you're on the right track and sense check what you're thinking.

Whichever approach you take, having cheerleaders to talk to who give you pep talks, who understand the fear and what you are going through and help you along the way is essential for dealing with all the day-to-day challenges we experience within our businesses.

Spend time on your planning and research

Planning and research form large part in developing confidence in your ability as a business owner.

Planning and research don't need to be scary or overly formal. Research is getting to know your students, the market, and what they need. When you know your students (existing or who you want to reach), you understand their needs and allow that knowledge to inform your plans. It becomes much easier for you to have confidence in what you are doing and why that is right for you and your business.

A plan is just that – an outline for how you're going to achieve your aim (like launching an online membership) and breaking down what needs to be done when, and how you're going to do it.

Simultaneously, you are less likely to succumb to a scarcity mindset because you know you are on the right track. You've invested the time, energy and effort into your research and planning; you know where you want to go and how to get there.

The boost to your confidence is big, and the scarcity and doubt melts away because you know what you're doing and exactly how that will benefit your students. This is what we are going to get into in the coming chapters in depth.

It will go wrong – that's business!

Yes, there will be hiccups. You'll try things and they won't quite work. You'll make mistakes. That's okay. It's part and parcel of owning a business and the sooner you get comfortable with messing up, the better.

All businesses have to revise plans, be agile and flexible and be prepared to change things along the way to get the desired result.

Get up, tweak it and go again! It's all part of running a business.

It takes time

Setting up a new online offering and growing it takes significant time as well as energy, determination and effort. This is not going to be the work of a few minutes. Like anything, it requires this investment.

Yes, you will get frustrated, have busier months and quieter ones, you will feel like you are shouting into the void at times and struggle with getting people across the line to joining and signing up. This might be further into the process or at the start. It's inevitable as part of the process as your students evolve on their journey and as you do as a teacher too. Time might need to be invested into diving into the issue, refining your Ideal Student, approach or messaging to get to the bottom of what is going on.

This is all part of the process and the sooner we are comfortable with this, the easier the process will become.

Mental health as a business owner

It would be remiss to not touch on mental health as a business owner in this section. Running a business is incredibly triggering at times, bringing up the mindset issues we've talked about already, causing incredible levels of stress. You might even be a person with anxiety or depression, trying to juggle those tricky conditions while finding your feet, and that is a thousand times more challenging.

My main advice here is you are a person running a business first and foremost. Not an entrepreneur who happens to be a person. That person (*you*) must come first always. If you aren't at your best, you aren't going to be able to deliver the best in your business either.

When your business is new, you're in a phase of growth or pivoting into something totally new it is so easy to get consumed by your work and end up working every hour in the day trying to get things moving and off the ground.

When you own a business there is always something to do, or someone who wants or needs something from you. Always. Most of these things can wait until another day.

Rest is so important to your wellbeing as a human and a business owner. I know you probably know this, especially if you teach yin or restorative yoga, but I guarantee you won't be practising what you preach to your students here.

Make sure you schedule rest in your work day. Set a start and finish time. Take a proper lunch break. Set aside time for regular tasks in your diary. Take days off. Start off with some strong boundaries – not replying to emails/messages outside hours you decide, turning your phone off, doing things you love.

All these things will help keep your stress down, help you feel aligned and keep on top of your wellbeing and mental health. If you feel like you need some support, reach out to a local provider, doctor or a charity for some additional support.

Remember, you're a human. You're also a business owner and you get to decide what feels good and what you do and don't want to do.

Chapter 3

STUDENT FIRST APPROACH

Putting Your Ideal Student's Needs at the Heart of Your Online Offering

In Chapter 2 we talked about each yoga teacher being different, offering a unique perspective and approach, and this concept extends to your business too.

When we are designing and planning a business it's important to think about what type of business you want to run, and therefore whose needs you'll be able to meet.

Each business will have a unique set of values that fall into what you do, how you do those things and the types of students you ultimately appeal to. Your students and your branding are two sides of the same coin and you can't work on one without the other.

There is no right or wrong when it comes to the mix of your business, what your online offering looks like, whether you create on demand classes or not, if you offer in-person classes as well. What will be great for the students of Teacher A won't be for Teacher B. What Teacher B does might work for Teacher C and Teacher A, and so on.

It's down to you to put your students first and design your offerings and brand around what their needs are and what resonates with them.

Whether you have existing students you want to bring on this journey, or you're starting afresh, there are a few key things to consider and some research to carry out which will help you shape your online offerings.

The foundations of your brand: what makes you the teacher you are

If you've bought this book, chances are you're a yoga, Pilates teacher or a personal trainer, meaning you are skilled in that role. That is one part of it and essential that you are certified and have the correct qualifications to carry out this kind of work.

Beyond this, you will have other skills, attributes or things about you that are transferable that all pull together to form your unique brand and help you appeal to specific groups of people.

You might be a gifted sportsperson, so you could find you're the perfect fit for teaching yoga targeted at people who participate in your sport. You might have a particular flair for boosting people's confidence and teaching in a super friendly, accessible way. All of these things are the essence and heart of your brand that attract students to you and your classes.

Our brand is way deeper than pretty colours or fonts, or a logo of a stick person sat in Lotus with a flower behind them. It's a feeling we get when we interact with a company or entity, uplifting, inspiring, seen and heard, educated. These are things that aren't necessarily tangible, and they require some thought and research to get right and be able to communicate effectively to reach, resonate and build relationships (plus sell) to our students.

Everything we do falls out of our branding: the type of students we attract through our marketing activities, the classes we teach and when, where and how we deliver them, the language we use, how we communicate with students, the social media channels we promote ourselves on.

At the root of this is understanding ourselves as yoga teachers and what our skills and strengths are.

A human story

Behind every business and huge corporation is a person who started it. That person has a life story, a journey and inspirations. Brands always use these stories as part of their branding and background.

People buy from people. People want to go on a journey from where they are to where they want to be.

When you share a bit of detail about who you are, what makes you tick, the journey you've been on, it helps people make a connection with you. If you've been on that journey, that's even better and that engages people straight away. When people are engaged and "warm", they're way more likely to buy from you. After all, people come to class with the teachers they click with and you being yourself helps them to figure out how you fit with them.

Maybe you've had an injury/illness, reduced corporate stress and found that yoga has helped you to do that, so you might naturally use this as a starting point for your online offering and talk about it whenever you can so you build rapport with people, so they think "they are like me".

Use your journey and inspirations to inform your branding and always keep sharing these things to help people to relate, know and trust you.

Your vibe and personality

Your personality and energy are hugely unique things. We all know some-one who is instantly likeable, has great energy and vibe to everything they do – and that's ultimately magnetic.

They uplift everyone around them and seemingly create positivity and magic with anything they do and work in a deeply authentic way. This comes from understanding who you are, confidence in your own skin and working with that authentically, being and teaching from the soul.

Just because you have a business doesn't mean you should hide it. As a yoga teacher you are the face and voice of your brand. It adds credibility, helps feed this authentic connection and builds likeability, which is key to getting people through the virtual door and bums on mats.

It can be a little bit cringy thinking about yourself like this and tough to actually pin down what the unique elements of your personality are, and super hard to do yourself. How you see yourself and how others see you and your qualities are often two different things.

There's a great exercise you can do with your family, friends, mentors, yoga teachers or trainee teacher pals, which will really help you get to the bottom of this:

Experience Your Uniqueness

Equipment needed: a marker, a pack of sticky notes/pieces of paper, a jar

1. Give all of these people a piece of paper or a sticky note and a pen.
2. Ask them to think of 3–5 adjectives that come to mind when

asked to describe your personality. Ask them to write each word on a separate piece of paper (so you have 3–5 different ones!).

3. Pop them in the jar.
4. Keep going until you've got a good selection from different people – people you are closer to, people who are friends, mentors and teachers.
5. Once you've done this, review what is in the jar.

This is a really fantastic way to experience how other people perceive you and can ultimately form the basis of your personal brand. It might give you an insight into the type of teacher you are and therefore the type of people who will resonate with you and be your Ideal Students.

A skill

You might have a skill that is a huge asset without realising that you have it.

If you're someone who has written, lectured or taught as part of a previous corporate career you might find you've got great experience in being able to explain complex concepts in a super clear way. You might be used to working in a public role dealing with large numbers of people and have developed a persona that puts people at ease instantly. If you are great at patient and clear explanation, nervous beginners might be an excellent student group to become your Ideal Students. A lot of these things are skills that people naturally have or have picked up over a long period of time doing a particular role and they are second nature.

This can also be quite a tricky thing to pin down yourself (because you possess the skills and might not appreciate them!) so you can use the previous exercise and ask the person to list 3–5 skills that you have.

Use Worksheet 3.1 to collate the qualities from both of the skill and personality exercises together in one place for easy reference. You'll be able to see all the common themes and traits at a glance. This will help anchor another one of the parts of your brand.

MY PERSONAL QUALITIES

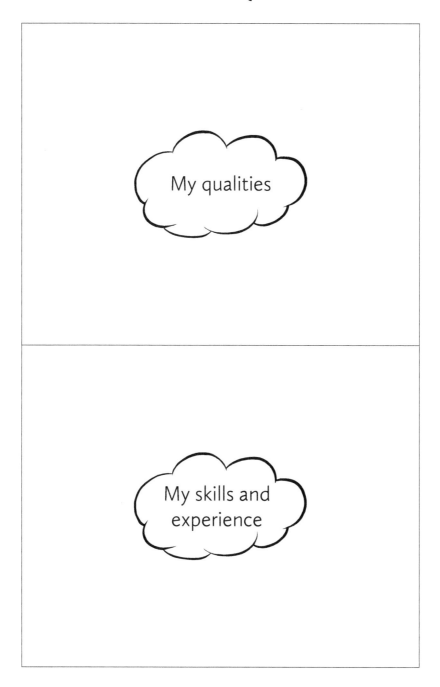

Bringing your brand to life

Once you've completed Worksheet 3.1 you can start bringing your brand to life using your answers to guide you along the process.

This stage is really fun but requires quite a lot of trial and error plus revisions to get to something that is perfect. Remember – it isn't for you, it's for your Ideal Student. It's great if you like it too, but it needs to be squarely focused at that student out there who wants a yoga teacher.

Step 1: Make a moodboard

Collate visuals and colour references together aimed at conveying your underpinning ethos and qualities to your Ideal Student. You can do this on Pinterest or on paper, whichever medium is your preference.

If you know your Ideal Student needs to blow off steam and doesn't take themselves seriously you might look for bright, fun images and branding examples and use those for your inspiration.

Equally you might fill your moodboard with empowering quotes if you know your Ideal Students have low confidence and need encouragement, or neutral calming images for students who need to reduce stress.

Step 2: The overall look and feel – fonts, colours and images

Once you've got your moodboard you can start to define and nail down your own unique interpretation of this for your brand.

I've outlined the stages and a top-level overview here. In reality, each stage happens in tandem and is tweaked until you get to a position where the overall look and feel is cohesive and sits well together and talks to that Ideal Student.

- Research fonts.
    - Pick fonts that are easily accessible or purchase a custom font just for you.
    - You'll want 2–3 – one for titles/headlines, one for subheadings and a contrasting easy-to-read font for body text.
- Research visual look and feel.
    - Research colour theory. Different colours have different effects and vibes, so look for colours that tie into how you want your Ideal Student to feel:
        » Want to cultivate calm? You might want to focus on natural images and earthy tones.

- » Want to bring fun? Use punchy brights and vibrant colours – bright pink, neons, orange.
- Start pulling a scheme of 5–7 colours together using the colour theory research. Coolors.co is my go-to for this, you can input a colour you like or leave it free and it will generate coordinating colour schemes.
- Research images and photography styles that give out the vibe that will attract your Ideal Students.
  - » Smiley, personable photography of you is accessible and puts people at ease.
- Logo design – this could be words or have an icon, or a mixture of the two.

Once you're happy, you can start to pull this together ready to use, with a little guide of what to use where, and set up some templates for you to use time and time again.

If this feels a bit overwhelming, I would really recommend investing in a brand consultant to help you with this. It's not super expensive, and it's a worthwhile investment. Design and branding is one of those things that looks really easy until you try and do it for yourself. It's a creative job that needs an artist's hand and often needs a deep understanding into marketing processes and journeys and how all the factors I mentioned above interact with each other.

So, if this isn't you, it's natural to feel a bit overfaced by this. If it really isn't your area of expertise research getting some help from a professional who has been recommended to you (not from fiverr or somewhere like that!). If there's a yoga teacher out there whose branding you love, you could ask them who they worked with and they would probably be quite happy to give you a recommendation.

It can also be quite time consuming and sometimes you are too close to your business to come up with something that truly resonates. This is another reason to outsource the job. There is nothing wrong with getting an external pair of eyes on what you've got so far and making it into a workable brand with top-notch visuals that will resonate with your Ideal Students.

This branding will grow and evolve over time as you do, so don't be afraid to revisit it when you feel it needs a refresh.

Video 4: Branding Basics can be downloaded from https://library.singingdragon.com/redeem using the voucher code JEWZDYR

Who are your students?

Students or clients are what your business exists to serve, whether that is a product like a pair of shoes or a service like a yoga class.

Once we understand what our strengths, skills and unique attributes are we can then think about who the people are this will resonate with before formulating our final branding and use this to inform the choices we make when we set up our online offerings.

So, who are your students or may want to be your students?

You may feel like this is really hard to do if you're starting out afresh without any students, but there is a way around this and it doesn't need to be a barrier.

Who is your Ideal Student?

Once we have an idea of what our attributes and skills are we can start to think about the type of person who would benefit from our business. These could be actual existing students or it could be hypothetical, the type of students you think your offering would resonate with.

In marketing land, Ideal Student Profiles/Avatars are traditionally used to do this. Ideal Student Profiles/Avatars are a detailed persona we create that fits the profile of one of our students – existing, or someone we want to be our student going forward. In the corporate world, these Profiles/Avatars have names, a detailed backstory with lots of information about the person, where they are in their journey, their socio-economic classification, the size of their house, how they think and act, the media they consume, age, level of free time, income level and so much more.

In reality, though, these aren't always the most helpful when it's just you in your wellbeing business. It can end up being really overwhelming to create in terms of time and energy, when actually a working format type document that isn't as formal or regimented is more than Good Enough for you to use in your business.

Teaching yoga or any class isn't a consistent experience either; we are continually evolving and shifting as teachers as our inspirations and influences develop. What we offer is a living, breathing and heart-led experience, not a simple product that is always exactly the same every time it is experienced. As we and our businesses grow and develop, we sometimes find these shifts mean that we are connecting with people we didn't expect to initially.

The other issue with Ideal Student Profiles/Avatars is their ability to create an atmosphere of exclusion. It is incredibly easy to create Ideal

Profiles that are pretty much identical to ourselves (or our internal view of ourselves), are very narrow and only attract others who are exactly like us, at the expense of the inclusion of other groups who would equally benefit from our offerings. It's very similar to an echo chamber – the people you attract are unconsciously mirrors of your values and beliefs and these biases get reinforced the more you hear the same things.

A really good example of this in action would be going to a yoga studio that seems to exclusively cater to thin white women in expensive leggings and wondering where all the diverse people represented in the local area are.

Essentially, our unconscious biases seep into our brand unintentionally and mean that we can end up not being able to help everyone who we could help because we're being tied to Ideal Student Profiles that are basically mirrors of ourselves.

All of this means we need to allow for this holistic flexing and growth within our Ideal Student Profiles, rather than using the more traditional rigid format used in the corporate world. It is still critical we have a view of who our students are, but it's time to be a bit savvier with how we do this.

The key thing is that we have some insight into these Ideal Students so we can get to know them, then design offerings that truly resonate with them that they want to purchase:

- Yoga and them: Are they aware of yoga? Have they thought about practising yoga and talked themselves out of it, have they tried and not found the right teacher, have they never thought about it, do they have misconceptions that make them think it's not for them?
- Social media: Are they present? Which channels do they like? Do they consume or interact? What will get them to interact? How much time do they spend there?
- Tech-savviness: Are they computer users regularly? Do they understand software? Do they prefer classes on computer or prefer to use a tablet?
- Media consumption: Do they read the local town paper or browse the local news or prefer to read magazines, national titles? Do they research their purchases on Google? Do they research on social media?
- How do we reach them? Are they more likely to respond to a flyer through their door or a post in their local Facebook group?

- What language resonates with them?
- What do they value? How do they purchase things? How do they interact with the world? What do they do for fun?

It doesn't matter how you go about doing this work, it's all about getting to know who you are actually wanting to talk to and attract to your business. There's nothing more annoying than posting about your membership platform or online classes and only getting other yoga teachers interact with your content, not the person you actually want to be seeing and buying from you.

Worksheet 3.2 will guide you through the process of getting to know and refine your Ideal Student Groups and their attributes and build this information into some loose profiles you can refer back to. One to three of these loose profiles is an ideal number. Too many and you spread yourself too thinly, too few and you could potentially be limiting your audience unnecessarily.

IDEAL STUDENT SUMMARY

Ideal Student Group:	

MINDMAP: Who are they? Where do they live? What do they enjoy doing? Hobbies? Complementary activities? What is their lifestyle like? What are their values?

Use this space to capture all the details about your Ideal Student Group. If you have more than one, use multiple sheets.

MINDMAP: What are their needs? What are their pain points related to yoga? Are there particular styles or things they need in their practice?

How can I meet those needs? What are the key themes?

MINDMAP: How do my Ideal Students want to feel when they interact with my business?

MINDMAP: How can I reach them?

What social media do they use (if any?), local publications, where do they spend time? Are there businesses they use I can partner with? Be creative!

Your research and analysis
Ask your students (existing or ideal)

If you have existing students, the best thing you can do is involve them in the process of creating your online offering: create a short survey and ask them what they'd like, what attracted them to your classes originally and why they keep coming. These are people who are already highly invested in what you do, so they are ready-made customers for your new offering and can help you refine what you do and who to target. Plus, everyone likes to have an input.

If you worry about getting participation and replies, you can explain why you are doing it and offer a small incentive prize draw like giving away a class to three randomly drawn participants. This encourages participation because there's something in it for the students potentially as well as helping you gain valuable knowledge.

Your students also feel valued, and it creates a wonderful community-led atmosphere around your business. It also leads to increased intent to buy because people are already invested in what you are doing.

Spending time getting to know and understand your students, asking for their input and building rapport go a really long way. It helps you develop not just the classes you teach but everything about how your students purchase and interact with you and your business, providing you with valuable insights into their behaviour – and the other people who fit the same Ideal Student Profile as your existing ones who you might be able to convert too.

If you don't have existing students, don't worry! You can still use this approach. You can find some yoga or local groups on Facebook and post a survey in there and get a more general opinion. You could also ask your peers and teacher trainers and get their input.

There are multiple free tools online that allow you to create surveys easily, like SurveyMonkey, or you can create your own using Google Forms or ask students to fill them in while they are waiting for you to start class. The methodology isn't important here; the data is the key part.

Research your Inspirational Figures

Inspirational Figures are the people you see out in the world who you look up to and think they're doing a great job. They don't necessarily have to be from the yoga world; they could be someone who has a particular attitude, energy or approach. The only rule is they have to inspire and uplift you and leave you with a positive feeling when you engage with them, their content, products or services.

We can all think of some big-name yoga teachers; really that isn't going to be the most helpful place to look for Inspirational Figures research purposes. Many of these teachers have significant resources in terms of funding, profile from social media and PR, teams of people working for them doing all the legwork. They are essentially the face and teacher of their brand with the support and help of everyone around them. Looking at this when you're starting out or researching your online offering isn't going to be constructive and could well trigger all kinds of issues we've been working on recognising and getting away from so far. It's not constructive because it can be literally like comparing apples and pears. Remember, what you see online isn't always a full and true account of what is really going on.

Instead, I'd suggest that you look at teachers with a similar profile or Ideal Student Profile to you as your Inspirational Figures. You may have a few teachers or business figures who offer an online presence that you think looks great or who teach in your local area and you might want to have a look at what they are doing, as well as understanding how and where they are talking to students who might be similar to those you are trying to reach.

By researching the market you can get an idea on what students appear to engage with, the price points, types and timings for classes and generally be inspired by the breadth of creativity that is out there in the field.

A word to the wise here – do not copy other teachers' work. Please. First, it's incredibly annoying and upsetting when someone does this to you and takes advantage of your hard work, energy and effort. Second, students see straight through it. Why? Because you aren't being authentically yourself. Who is the only person who can do you? You are. That's your superpower.

Finally, it's theft. Copyright infringement is a very serious crime that can lead to hefty fines and jail time if it is proved you did it. So... just don't.

Absolutely see what is out there as part of your market research, note down the common points, how they seem to be landing with the people in your Ideal Student Group, and then develop your own offering, position and brand to suit.

What is going to make buying from you easy?

Another reason we want to get to the bottom of how our students want to interact with our business is that we want to make it pleasurable and easy for them to spend money with us and make that journey of decision to buying as smooth and easy as possible.

Picture this. You're in a room that is full of barriers. You want the chocolate cake that is on the other side of the room, but to get it…you've got to climb over all the barriers. I certainly couldn't be bothered with that; it's irritating, and I don't want the cake that much.

That's what buying from you could be like if you have a really convoluted, multi-step, fiddly process. Would this put you off?

1. Student emails teacher for a space in class, waits for reply.
2. Teacher emails back – says yes, books the student in on a spreadsheet/notebook, replies to confirm the space and asks for payment.
3. Student accepts space and sends teacher the payment.
4. Teacher waits for payment, then notes down that they've been paid. Sends student a manual email with any information for class and forms needed.
5. Student receives and completes forms and emails them back.
6. Teacher receives forms, reviews and then files away.

I'm betting the answer is probably.

Sometimes this occurs in a yoga business that started as a once a week class and that system does work initially. What tends to happen is the business grows, the owner doesn't see the need to invest in systems and processes because what they're doing works, so why change it, and also because of fear of the size of that investment.

But once people have been put off, that is it. They are far less likely to want to purchase from you again, because they've already had a negative interaction with your business.

Everything you do as a business owner isn't for you. It's for your students.

It doesn't matter if it causes you a bit more admin time to put your classes on an online system. In fact, systems like this save significant time once they're up and running and you are confident using them. Also, people are more likely to buy again and again so you actually end up bringing more money in with less active involvement from you.

It matters that your student can book a place for a class in a few minutes, pay using their bank card, get an email confirmation and reminder plus any relevant information straight to their inbox.

It's about them having a great experience and ultimately, great experiences = happy students = more recommendations plus existing students buying more from you.

The system and approach that you choose will be informed by what your student's tech-savviness is like – are they okay with having a phone app only? Do they need something super simple? Do they trust PayPal or paying with a card online?

These are all considerations we make during the process of designing our online offerings, informed by our Ideal Student Profile research.

Bringing all the research together

Once you've spent some time working through the worksheets provided so far, you'll have all the information you need to move on with developing your online offering.

You might have chosen to read first and then complete the worksheets, or completed them as you have gone through the first section of the book.

The best advice I can give you here is to make sure you've spent the time researching. This research will inform the decisions you're going to make in the next section of the book, when we move on to *the how*.

Chapter 4

THE HOW

Ways to Teach Online: Live and On Demand Options

As teachers, we are used to teaching live and face to face only. If you're not in class you've missed the experience and online opens up our options exponentially.

There are lots of different ways to teach online and that can be really overwhelming, even when you've done all the pre-work we've done together so far.

In this chapter, we're going to get down to business. We're going to talk through the different ways to teach online, the pros and cons of all the options that are available to us, then get down to deciding how to go about getting ourselves teaching online in a way that works for our Ideal Students.

Live classes

Live classes are the closest format to our traditional way of teaching; we teach a class at a certain time on a certain platform. This is an active form of income and requires our direct involvement to make it happen.

The pros and cons of live classes

Having a set schedule of live classes is great for students as it helps create a routine for practice and accountability because the class is happening at a specific time and place. There's a wonderful community aspect too, as you might choose to have a pre- and post-class chat with those who would like to take part. Teaching a live class online is a familiar format to our traditional model, delivering a group class to a screen with everyone present rather than face to face. You are able to give feedback in real time to your class and help them on a deeper level because you can interact with them. It's really convenient for you as a teacher as you don't need lots of set up or travel time, and the same for your students too. Live classes have a lower entry point for you as a teacher because the equipment needed and investment in time to learn new skills is lower, making it a great way to dip your toes in the water.

The downside of any online offering is that not every student is going to want to participate in an online world. Busy households, lack of space and confidence with technology can prevent students from participating. The requirement for a decent internet connection and a device capable of accessing the internet can also be a barrier. If your students live rurally and rely on a satellite internet connection or are in a low-income household, they might not have access to a broadband connection, a laptop or tablet to join with.

Even if we try really hard, the experience online is slightly different and not everyone is going to like that. Other issues in the online space are the pricing models offered by businesses who have scale on their side and the student understanding of the value of a live class versus picking a random class on YouTube.

PROS	CONS
• Routine for students • Convenient for you and the student • Set time for practice • Familiar teaching style for you • Students get feedback • Community aspect • Easier to get started – less equipment required and fewer new skills to learn	• Online isn't for every student – busy house/lack of space/routine • Isn't identical to in-person experience • Low prices in marketplace • Student perception of value of live classes • Internet and device use to access class

Teaching live classes: methods and considerations
There are several different routes for live classes, falling into the categories of interactive and streamed.

INTERACTIVE
Interactive classes offer the benefit of two way engagement. Students can see and hear you, and you can see them. Students can interact with you via

written messages or by talking to you directly when they need additional support or have questions.

This is the closest experience to being in an in-person class we can offer online. It is much easier to convert students to an experience that they are familiar with, rather than something that is totally new to them, like on demand classes.

The most popular method for delivering interactive classes is via video conferencing or calling software. Providers like Zoom have absolutely boomed over recent years; it is important to note that Zoom isn't the only option if you want to deliver interactive live classes.

A slightly less conventional method would be to use a platform like FaceTime or WhatsApp, which is also an accessible option for many people that doesn't require extra technology. I'd suggest that these options are better suited for any online 1:1s rather than a group class scenario.

Google Meet, Microsoft Teams, GoToMeeting or similar providers also have platforms that might be better suited to group classes for your students and their specific needs. They might be really user friendly, which is ideal for those who aren't tech confident, or allow people with hearing loss to have the option to closed caption your teaching in real time at their end. You might have access to a software with your email account that would work well without having to pay any extra. When it comes to decision time, we want to bear all these factors in mind.

A lot of online booking software providers (which we will come on to in depth in the next chapter) offer integrations with different video conferencing software. This is an absolute godsend and saves you so much time, effort and energy which frees you up to get on with teaching and planning whilst cutting down your admin time significantly. Some booking systems integrate fully with your conferencing software and will create a link for the class for you and make that visible when a student has booked and paid. Others will have a space for you to drop a link that you've created in instead. Depending on the number of classes you are teaching and how much or little admin you want to do, you might elect to research your booking system and live class software in tandem and decide on both elements together.

STREAMING

Live streaming is anything where students can only see and hear you, and you cannot hear or see them. Students might be able to interact and comment via a chat box if this feature is enabled during the stream but the level of back and forth in terms of your ability to observe and feed back on what you can see when compared to an interactive class isn't there.

Popular methods include:

- Instagram Live – on your page or a private member only page
- stream on YouTube – private or public stream
- private Facebook group – paid members group or on your page
- stream on your own website
- stream via a yoga platform.

The streaming method is more complex for yoga teachers and requires a bit more thought and process behind the set up. The first consideration is payment. When we stream freely on our own Instagram pages, anyone on Instagram can see that stream, even if they don't follow us. If the class we are teaching is part of a paid offering, this is something we obviously don't want to happen. You might well choose to teach a mini free, streamed practice as a taster to market your online offering, which is a different conversation. Some platforms like Facebook offer the facility to create in platform paid events, while others, like Instagram, don't have this facility at the time of writing for business accounts.

How do we go about ensuring people who have paid have access and know where the class is being streamed? Do they need to follow a private account? Be added into a private group? Do we need to remove people who haven't paid? All these things create an additional layer of admin and processes to develop. To allow us to be able to manage all these extra considerations, we might make our offering less flexible and offer monthly access only. This may suit some student groups incredibly well, but not others.

Are your students on the platform you want to stream on or social media in general? It's no good deciding you want to stream on Facebook when most of your students don't have an account or don't want one! It adds a big hurdle in the way of their decision to purchase. If you are keen on streaming only, investigating some of the options offered by website providers like Wix, that allow you to stream directly from your own website, these could be a better fit.

The quality of the product can also be variable. Platforms like Facebook and Instagram often reduce the size of live stream videos and audio quality in comparison to video conferencing software providers. For simple things like guided meditation this might be okay, but for a class with lots of movement having clarity issues with the audio and juddery, pixelated video is going to compromise the student's enjoyment and experience and your ability to charge for the classes.

Looking at this from a student's perspective, is the streaming experience different enough to buying an on demand offering? The value in live classes is the amount of feedback and interaction given. Depending on the student group, they might much prefer a live interactive option instead of a streamed class.

For some students, streaming is a great option. Many students experience anxiety around being visible online in a class and don't feel comfortable turning their camera off when everyone else has theirs on. For them the streaming experience where they can see and hear only you and they can participate without the worry of being seen or heard is a benefit.

Many insurers also require that we keep accurate records of who is in each class in case of any cases lodged against us. That is impossible to do if we are streaming via Instagram or Facebook to a global audience, but very easy to do teaching a private class on video conferencing software. Some insurers are happy to cover online classes in all formats continuously now that the concept has proved to be successful; others require full records, capped class sizes and an individual consultation with each student; others charge additional premiums depending on the methods you use to teach your classes. It is important to understand how you can meet these requirements when you are teaching online no matter which methods you ultimately settle on, and what your own insurers' requirements are.

USING AN ONLINE STUDIO PLATFORM

There are also a number of platforms emerging currently, such as Kuula TV, that offer a dedicated platform for your live classes while also taking care of payments and scheduling in one place. It's a similar experience to being a teacher under the banner of a studio but being able to charge and set your own prices rather than being paid a set fee.

The commercial terms each site operates on are slightly different; some charge a larger or smaller percentage, some allow you to own your student's data, some do not. Some have their own proprietary technology for interactive classes and allow students to record the class, others allow you to switch facilities on and off depending on what you want for your own offering.

If you are an independent teacher, you might want all your students on your website booking their classes and practising on demand as, after all, the longer people spend on your site, the more valuable it looks to the Google gods and the higher it ranks when people are searching.

If you are someone who teaches a class or two each week around another job, the draw of having such minimal admin and being on a platform with a larger audience therefore being visible by a larger number of students would be a big bonus.

On the flipside, if there are numerous teachers on that platform with wildly different rates, does this mean the teachers who charge low fees have monopoly and therefore feed the commoditisation of yoga issues we discussed in Chapter 2? I don't have an answer for this one at the moment, as it is such a new arena of operation at the time of writing. If this is an approach you may be interested in then I suggest you do a lot of research into this, tread carefully and take time to research the pros and cons of each individual platform and how they operate.

INTERACTIVE
Two Way Engagement You teach, they participate, you give feedback
• Zoom
• Google Meet
• Microsoft Teams
• GoToMeeting
• Skype
• Online studio platforms – Kuula, Ribbon Experiences
• FaceTime • WhatsApp

STREAMED
One Way Engagement You teach, they participate, no feedback or very limited via one way short comments, not conversational
• Instagram Live
• Private Facebook group
• Your Business Facebook page
• Your website/Wix Streaming (if you have a Wix website)
• Online studio platforms

On demand classes

On demand is the catch-all term for any pre-recorded or pre-prepared content that you make available to your students which they can participate in anytime, anywhere, without you physically having to be present or engaged in the process.

The pros and cons of on demand classes

On demand is a huge opportunity for yoga teachers as it provides us with a passive stream of income on an ongoing basis. As I mentioned in Chapter 1, this is essential for diversifying our income and having more than one way to earn money in our businesses. Passive income is ideally suited for recurring payment options like memberships or subscriptions, meaning students pay us continually for access to our on demand offerings. They don't have to remember to pay, which is super convenient for them, and we get paid time and time again for work we did weeks or months ago, and don't have to spend time or energy chasing payments, which is a huge win for us too.

It's also absolutely fantastic for students with busy lives, as they aren't restricted to a timetabled class and can practise with you at any time they like. On demand classes also aren't restricted to students in our time zone or local area only; anyone with internet would be able to practise with you, no matter where they are.

There are always students in our existing student base who would love on demand classes. It means they can practise with you more frequently and they don't miss out when you go away. It's feasible that you can actually end up with more income from each student because of it, if you design your offering in a clever way that offers wide and flexible access.

It's also an economy of scale. Quite often we can offer on demand packages at a lower cost than our in-person classes because the overheads are so much lower and the number of people joining in is effectively limitless. It also allows us to reach students who have lower incomes and offer an option for them to get involved in yoga at an affordable price point.

Because students aren't in a live class environment, they aren't getting real time feedback from you that is personalised and the community aspect of chats before and after class isn't easy to replicate, depending on the model you choose to operate with.

This isn't the end of the world, though, as there are ways we can create an online community as part of our offering. Creating a private forum on our Members Area, or a private Facebook group, a monthly Q&A call or catch up are all wonderful ways to bring the community spirit to life.

The downsides are a lot of the same ones as live classes: not every student is going to want to practise in this way. Practising on demand is also challenging for a lot of people because there isn't a regimented time to do it, it's there for them to do as and when they want, and having self-accountability and motivation to roll your mat out when you'd rather be sitting drinking tea and watching Netflix is a real struggle.

Another issue is the proliferation of full-length classes on YouTube. It's really hard to convince students to part with money for an online on demand practice when you have previously put full-length classes on You-Tube. Your classes are the product you make your income from and this is why I don't advocate putting things you can make money from on YouTube.

Even if you don't post full-length practices to YouTube, there are millions of other yoga teachers out there making this choice in the hope they grow their audience to a huge size where they qualify for monetisation (1000 subscribers and 4000 view hours per year at the time of writing) and that flow class just isn't enough of a differentiator anymore. It's very much like standing and screaming into the void. The question I would get you to ask is this – does this shift the needle in my business? In most cases, no. Posting your 60-minute flow won't help you get paying customers; you'll only end up with people who aren't your Ideal Student taking advantage and demanding more freebies.

There isn't the appreciation out there in the yoga-consuming world that every time someone takes a class with [Insert YouTube Yogi Here] that teacher makes money because the student watched an ad before their class.

It's not worth trying to compete with the YouTube yoga juggernauts out there. We need to think about what we can offer that is uniquely us – what sets us apart – that our Ideal Students will resonate with.

On demand is also a lot more intensive in terms of time, equipment and skill level. You're going to need camera equipment, lighting and SD cards to film the class with. You're also going to need time to set up the space and equipment, film the class, film any corrections or fix mistakes, edit the class footage and upload it to a video hosting platform before anyone can do anything with it. There is a learning curve, especially when you start.

I'm pleased to say it does get easier with time but, being real with you, it can be a right pain in the backside sometimes. Some days you go to film it doesn't happen because of tech issues, you being tired or whatever else. And that is okay.

PROS	CONS
• Convenient for you • Convenient for the student • Passive and recurring revenue into your business • Film once and done • Larger potential audience	• Online isn't for every student – busy house/lack of space/routine • Isn't identical to in-person experience • Internet and device use to access class • No feedback and harder to nail the community aspect • Higher skill level, more equipment and technique to record classes, edit and have platform to share them • Value proposition – "Why should I pay when I can YouTube for free?"

Ways to teach on demand classes

There are a number of different ways to offer on demand classes which should again be chosen according to how your Ideal Student would want to consume your classes.

A common approach is a Yoga membership. This is a website (dedicated or a restricted area on your website) that holds access to a range of practices only available to members. A membership is absolutely flexible to whatever you want to include, and you can be as creative as you like. You might choose to teach classes on their own, offer meditations, downloads, forums, workshops or nidras, offer access to discounts, live classes in any format, a single price point or a tiered system of benefits at different price points. The world is really your oyster here.

There are also community-based platforms like Patreon, which are membership community sites specifically designed for this purpose. Generally offering practices on platforms like this attracts a significantly higher fee than creating your own offering.

Using a platform like Patreon is a great option for those with limited time and resources, but at the expense of search engine optimisation (SEO) benefits of being on your own platform under your own branding in a similar way to the Online Yoga Studio Platforms we discussed earlier.

You could also elect to rent or purchase single classes or class bundles for a specified period or in perpetuity. Permanent purchases would be offered at a higher price point, and single classes could be offered for much less.

If you taught an online workshop live, you could record it and make it available afterwards so it becomes something you can continue to earn from on an ongoing basis.

You might also elect to design a course running for a designated period – 4, 6 and 12 weeks are popular periods – and offer these as a self-paced course via a course provider like Teachable, Kajabi or on your own platform, or there's also the option to run these as live and interactive sessions.

Taking a blended approach: a mix of live and on demand content

There is also the option to offer a bit of everything through a mixture of live and on demand content either individually or as a package or to offer both options. Your Ideal Students then have a range of different online products to choose from at different price points, which gives you a higher chance of converting them.

It is worth thinking about this initially and what that would look like for you and your business, even if you decide to add this into your offering further down the line. This means you are set up with a pricing approach that is fit for purpose and you don't have to reinvent the wheel if and when you do decide to expand your range of online products.

A membership is a great place to do this. Memberships can be flexed up and down with tiers being added or tweaked to reflect your business over time.

You might elect to start off with a single tier offering a choice of on demand classes only for a lower price point, then expand it to offer some live classes within a higher price point or offer a flat fee with a set number of live classes each week.

You might offer live classes on a pay as you go basis and offer a membership tier that includes live online classes and access to on demand content too.

The other benefit of working with a membership model with live classes included is you are creating a recurring income and being paid for those classes, versus a traditional timetabled class where people buy and pay each week and you have a fluctuating level of income. You may still want to offer that as an option so that you are offering choice as well as maximising your level of income from each of your classes.

A course might offer on demand classes and some interactive discussion sessions covering the course material for that particular week.

Making a decision

It might seem really tough to make a decision because there are so many different approaches and ways to teach online. I've included a few ideas throughout this chapter in the relevant sections to give you an idea of what is out there.

The decision to get to at this point is about the *how*. Do you want to teach live online classes, live stream classes or on demand? The exact mechanics of how you go about doing this will take a little bit of time to research and develop.

It is totally okay to start off with one thing. Live online classes are the simplest option to get up and running; an on demand membership is more complex. You might elect to start simple and develop the other bits for launch later on once you're happy and have spent some time on it. It is totally flexible and can be changed as and when needed as you start to explore this space.

The good news is that there is no right or wrong answer or one single way of doing this. There is probably more than one way to do this for your Ideal Students too. You might start with one idea and refine it as you go as your students' needs also change and evolve.

The starting point is thinking about your students (ideal or existing) and what offerings are going to suit them initially.

If your Ideal Student would be interested in live classes, it is important to get an idea of the times of day or days they are wanting to practise and for how long. A common trend amongst students is the need for shorter classes, around 30–45 minutes, rather than a full 60–90-minute practice when they are practising at home. They might also practise more frequently and want a wider variety of classes.

A consideration that isn't immediately obvious is how all of this works for you as a teacher, fitting in online classes to your schedule. This can be a little bit of a headache. It is way more tiring to teach online. Students are relying on you for visual feedback, so you might have to demo a lot more than you may be used to. Some students learn by watching, others by listening. You'll have people quite literally standing there watching you and if you don't move...they won't either! They'll have pinned you to their screen and won't have any visual references other than you (even if it is as simple as "arms overhead"). It's important to consider your own energy and health in this decision as well, as teaching a full live online and in-person schedule isn't sustainable long term and could well land you in the physiotherapist's office with loads of niggles.

It is really tough to teach a live online class at the same time as teaching an in-person class to a high level, even before you factor in logistical challenges like sufficient internet, space for all the equipment to teach online and background noise. It's worth considering your timetable and seeing how and where you can facilitate both options either at the same time or separately and adapting your schedule to a manageable level so you've got some options to choose from.

Another consideration is how your students are likely to behave. Are they going to want to attend an online class then practise on demand on a day you aren't teaching? Or are they going to come to in-person classes only? Understanding how your students (ideal or existing) are likely to behave will allow you to set up your timetable to accommodate as many of these groups as possible and increase your income.

You may find some students happily float around all your different offerings – joining online, coming in person and practising on demand. Others might only ever practise online or come in person and need some seriously strong persuasion to deviate from this. You might think they'll do one thing then they behave completely differently in reality and you need to tweak your plans to meet this need you hadn't anticipated. That's all good and part of the process.

Your approach to capturing these students is likely to vary too and you might also want to explore ways of getting each of these student groups engaged with the parts of your offering they aren't currently taking part in.

To get more people trying out more of the different parts of your online offering you could do an option that allows access to everything you do at a great price point. It would need to be something that offers mega flexibility, choice and be a no-brainer for students to sign up to. It could be a sale month where you offer unlimited online and on demand classes or a package that offers a bit of everything available all the time. You could also offer an annual membership at a sale price at launch. When these offers are time limited people are more inclined to purchase them.

The students you already have in your classes are your hottest leads. They're already customers of yours and therefore it is much easier to convince them to join your online offerings. They've bought in to you and your ethos and love your classes. It's much easier and less costly in terms of time and resource to convert someone like this than someone off Instagram who has never heard of you before. That Instagram yogi has to go on a heck of a journey to get to the same place as someone who comes to your classes week in and week out and wishes they could do more classes with you.

On demand offers you the space to do some different things that you normally wouldn't be able to do, like mini workshops, trainings, chats and sharing about wider yoga culture, and provide added value way beyond what the world of YouTube has to offer.

What else can you offer that your students can't get anywhere else? Maybe there is something that you know in depth that you can add? Is there something any existing students ask you about regularly? Do you have a signature workshop offering that you could break into chunks and create?

There are so many things you can do and so much creativity you can exploit with how you get teaching online. It allows you to create something uniquely you and that is so amazing.

You won't have all the answers right away, you might even feel a bit overwhelmed by choice. I recommend taking a bit of time to go away, digest this section and revisit in a few days.

Concentrate on one thing initially if you want to launch quite quickly; if you are happy to take a little bit of time on this your offering could be a wider one. It really is up to you.

Pricing: charging your worth and how to figure that out

We've talked about the importance of fair and ethical pricing that allows you to make a liveable wage throughout the book so far, which is all well and good – but you need to know *how* to do that.

Charging your worth isn't about plucking a number out of thin air and using that as your price. No, no, no. It's about getting to a pricing strategy and plan that feels right, it's founded in research and takes your own experience, costs and earnings into account. Fair doesn't automatically mean high, either – it means fair and evidence based.

There's no way I can give a hard and fast figure here as to what constitutes too little, other than if it is under minimum wage when you split the fee out into hours taken to do the job then that's of course too little. Every yoga business is different and it is up to you to do the research and invest some time in developing a policy that works for you.

Step 1: Research

First, you need to research prices that are out in the marketplace for classes/memberships that are similar to the one you're interested in launching.

Spend some time having a google, looking what is out there in the marketplace and what the prices are and what is included for that. You also need to take contextual information into this – is this a studio's offering, an independent teacher with a huge platform or a teacher who is more experienced and established?

Drop all of this information into a spreadsheet and sort it, price lowest to highest, duplicate the information and remove all the teachers who aren't in the same contextual situation as you.

If you are a new teacher or launching something new, your price point is going to be at the lower end of the banding. You don't want to undercut, you want to be at a competitive and comparative point.

As you get confident in people gaining value in the offering and your skill and ability to sell grows over time, you can then look to increase prices or add more expensive tiers into the offering too.

Step 2: Your commercials

You need to get a handle on what your overheads are. Overheads are your costs: things like insurance and the initial investment in equipment to carry out your work.

Once you know that you'll have a minimum amount you'd need to make from each class or from your membership. Any business needs to break even and meets its cost as a bare minimum.

Then you can look to add your wages on top. You need an understanding of the time investment you need to make to create the offering – the time to teach the class, deal with admin, payments, students and everything else.

Once you've got that you can then look to split this across the number of students you think you can get signed up.

Step 3: Spread of options and price points

Ideally you want to have a range of options and choices for people: drop in for weekly bookings, block booking discounts for regular students and so on. You might also want to have a membership that has a cheaper entry point, a middle and a top level.

What you have where and when will entirely depend on how you want to work and build your offering over time.

Worksheet 4.1 will help you rough out your online offering and the price points that feel good for you. Use as many copies of this sheet as you need to get to a fully mapped out range of options.

THE HOW: MY OFFERINGS

Type	☐ Live Classes ☐ On Demand	☐ Streamed ☐ Rental ☐ Individual sale	☐ Interactive ☐ Bundle (for sale) ☐ Membership
Order of Introduction	1. 2. 3.		Rough launch: Rough launch: Rough launch:

LIVE CLASSES								ON DEMAND		
Type/length								Single price membership Tiered membership	☐ . . . . ☐ Tiers . . . . ☐ from . . . . ☐ to	
Day/ time	M	T	W	T	F	S	S	Tier 1 Price	Name: . . . . Content	

PRICING	Single	☐	Tier 2 Price	Name: . . . . Content	
	Sliding scale	☐			
	Class passes	☐			
	Membership	☐	Tier 3 Price	Name: . . . . Content	
DELIVERY METHOD	Platform and student journey:				
			Single rentals	☐	
			Sale	☐	
STUDENT PROCESS	How do students, book, pay and view?				
			Bundles	☐ Price: . . . . Content	

Chapter 5

THE ESSENTIALS

Goal Setting, Planning, Processes and Systems

Goals, plans, processes and systems are not sexy. But they are so essential in any business. This is why this chapter is called *The Essentials*! These are the things that help you get clear on what you're doing, how you're going to deliver it and what you need to do it. These are the things that make everything you do work – this is the vehicle you use to get your yoga out to the world. None of it would happen without having a goal, plans in place on your side of things or processes and systems for students to use.

In this chapter we will be covering the knowledge you need to set yourself some goals, how to plan what you want to do, then diving into websites, booking systems, member areas, how we go about getting paid and video editing software.

Goal setting: the big picture piece

Goal setting isn't as complex as the corporate world would have you believe. Goals are statements that help you to get from where you are to where you want to be over a defined period of time.

The most common method of setting goals is the SMART method:

S	Specific
M	Measured/measurable
A	Achievable
R	Realistic
T	Timebound

Each goal should be specific, for instance, launch my first online flow class. Measured or measurable involves the design of how you know that goal is hit or not. Something like a class is really easy – is it happening or not would be your measure. Some goals could be financial or member driven, therefore you'd need to have a numerical measurement for a goal like this.

Achievable and realistic are what I like to refer as sense checks rather than for inclusion in the wording of your goal. To create and build a whole new website, film and edit five classes and put them on sale in one day wouldn't be doable and is really unrealistic too. But if you gave yourself two months to do that, it would certainly satisfy both of these criteria.

Each goal should have a timeframe that is specific, achievable and realistic given the scale of the goal and the work involved to make it happen. You'll most likely have a series of goals that are shorter term (sub 6 months), medium term (12 months) and long term (3, 5 and 10 years). You might want to start with a list of goals and then prioritise these depending on cost, scale of project and required resources and use this to set your timeframes.

You can also write your goal in first person using an *I Will* or *I Am* statement. This doesn't always apply for a larger business, but when it is just you flying solo in your business it is a great thing to do (for extra points you can even drop this onto your vision board so it is front and centre every day).

Here are some examples:

- I will launch an online membership in six months time.
- I will run a marathon next summer.
- I am going to grow the number of clients on my membership from 0 to 1000 in two years.

Once we have our goal defined, we can then start thinking about making this into a plan, and the first stage here is breaking down the milestones that need to happen along the way to deliver the goal.

If you want to launch a membership, that might be something like:

- Plan launch date.
- Set test date.
- Create first set of content for the membership.

Once you have the key milestones noted down, these get broken down even further into our plan.

Worksheet 5.1 is here to help you through the process of setting your goals and milestones.

Take some time jotting down a few goals. You'll probably find you have more that fall into the short and medium term categories, and 1–2 in the long term category. Use one copy of Worksheet 5.1 per goal, downloading and using as many copies as you need.

GOAL SETTING AND MILESTONES

What do I want to achieve?		
How am I going to measure it?	☐ Yes/No (did it happen?) ☐ Numerical (X to Y/ financial) ☐ Sentiment (feelings based)	What are the specifics of the measurement? Add the detail here (i.e. 10 members in 3 months)
Timeframe	☐ Short ☐ Medium ☐ Long	Is this achievable and realistic? ☐ Yes ☐ No (revise)

My goal statement

Milestones and progress tracker Identify the key steps and stages to meeting your goal, write them in below. Track your progress on the right hand columns.	Started	In progress	Complete

Your plan

If you imagine goals as the scenery in a painting, your plan is the bit that adds the pretty flowers and the colour onto that canvas.

Business plans are another thing that sounds super scary but they don't need to be formal and are quite often something we do without even thinking about it. Letting you in on a secret, you've been making a business plan throughout this book without even knowing it...sneaky, I know.

A plan is simply all the research into the market, Ideal Customers/ Students, what their needs are, options for the product/s or offering/s that meet their needs, the details of each offering, then the steps and things that need to happen to bring it to life, with some goals as the starting point – taking this from something on paper into reality. A plan often has smaller plans within it, like Russian nesting dolls – a marketing or launch plan or a financial forecast.

When everything is down on paper it is easy to see what needs to be done. When you do this process over a few days or weeks, you will naturally think of more things that need to be done and it gives you a complete overview of every little thing that needs to be considered, the order when things need to happen and where you could potentially look to get some help with what you want to do.

I know outsourcing is a tough decision because it is very chicken and egg. You need the help, but the money isn't coming in so you can't afford it, but you don't have the time to build things because you're too busy doing rather than driving things forward. I get it, I've been there. It isn't easy.

The best piece of advice I can give here is, if you're wondering if it's the right time to get some help, it's probably the right time. If it doesn't quite feel like that, it is 100 per cent a balancing act – if you are looking at your plan and it is overwhelming you and you're not sure if you can do it – ask these questions:

- Can the timeframe be extended?
- Can the offering be made more manageable? Could you design the offering so there's less content to produce – release one class a week instead of needing five ready all at once for an on demand membership?
- Can you get some help on a skill swap? You could get some help from a virtual assistant or coach in exchange for delivering yoga lessons for them potentially?

- Are there any grants you can get from the local council or authority? There are lots of grants available for start-ups or small businesses from a variety of sources. It's worth doing some research and asking local government for a signpost to who might be able to support you.

You also need to allow for some wiggle room in your timeframe. Any time you are learning new skills, testing new platforms or tech or working with others there is bound to be some slippage. It will take you a lot longer to figure out how to do things the first time you do them – you might need to go back to the drawing board on your tech and research another platform or someone doing a job for you might have an emergency and deliver late. It also helps you keep your stress levels under control by removing some self-imposed pressure and creates space for you to breathe.

It's not the end of the world if you get to fleshing out your plan and ultimately things need to be tweaked. Remember it's your business, so you can do what you want, and it is *so* much better to know this before you get started and into the process of creating the offering.

Your plan can be done in any form that suits you. You might want to start on paper with a brain dump of all the milestones, the tasks that would need to be done to complete that milestone using Worksheet 5.2: Project Planner (coming up in a moment). Then you could transfer all of this into a digital format for easy manipulation, tracking status of your project and recording who is doing what task. You could use a Google Sheet, or you might want to have a look at using a collaborative tool like Asana, Trello, Basecamp or Teamwork. Or you could keep it purely on paper, or digitally. It is entirely down to you and what works best for you.

PROJECT PLANNER

Task	Due by	Resources needed	Who	Status			Notes
				Started	In progress	Complete	

Once we've got our plan in place we can get on with bringing it to life. To do that, we are going to need some resources, processes and systems.

Why do I need processes and systems?

- They save you time:
  - less admin – no more booking people in on paper or a spreadsheet
  - clear process – less time on emails and correspondence asking questions
  - students book and pay – no time wasted chasing payments.
- They take you out of active involvement and make you money without you having to be there, so you can work on your business rather than being in it all the time.
- They remove hurdles for your students and make it easier for them to spend more with you (remember "what's going to make buying from you easy" from Chapter 3? Literally...processes and systems!).
- They allow you the capacity to scale and expand what you're doing easily.

Your website

If you are a teacher who wants to build an online offering (that's why you're reading this book!) you *need a website* of your own. Not an Instagram page with thousands of followers. No, no, no...

A website is your own corner of the internet. You want to get your followers over on your own website which is your digital house and have them signing up to your site and newsletter. The more they're on there, reading blogs, booking and taking classes the better for you. The Google gods love it and push you higher up the pages.

So much emphasis is put on the importance of Instagram/other social media platforms and building a community there at the expense of your own space on the internet. The problem is, Instagram and social media is rented real estate. You could lose your account, and then what are you going to do? Exactly. Shift part of your focus to creating your own space, nurturing your people and getting them over to your own corner of the internet.

If you have direct contact with your Ideal Students, you can build relationships, trust and sell to them and they're infinitely warmer than someone who hangs out watching us on Instagram.

The idea is that your website does the work for you rather than you having to continuously field the same questions time and time again (although be prepared – you will still get people messaging you asking for information that is clearly on your website. Especially if they've found you on Facebook!). People sometimes want to be fed the answer. Quite often, these people who take up lots of energy and time don't ever convert. Overall, though, this saves you a lot of time dealing with unnecessary admin and enquiries as people who are engaged are way more likely to carry out a good amount of research.

Websites are often seen as a vastly expensive thing and yes, they can be, for something built from the bare bones upwards. It doesn't need to be this way for what you'll need as a yoga teacher. The requirements for a yoga website are simple and anyone a little bit tech savvy will be able to make something themselves that'll do the job over the space of a day or so. If you're not confident you can easily hire someone to set it up for you for a reasonable price as a package along with your brand design.

The bare minimum: what we definitely need

- Home page – a page to direct people around your website. A short welcome, what you do overview, about you, reviews (ask for some!). You might also want a section where you can highlight workshops or special offers here.
- Classes page – a single page covering the style of your classes, FAQs, who they're suitable for, descriptions, link to booking and timetable. Depending on what you offer you could have extra pages explaining your pricing, 1:1s or any corporate packages you offer under a menu.
- Booking system.
- Contact information.
- Newsletter sign up.

Building a good website

I'm not going to lie: building a good website is a bit of an art. Luckily there are plenty of tools to help and I'm going to share some of my tips here too.

Your website is your digital shop window and a real reflection of you and your brand. When potential students visit your site, it is crucial that you capture their attention very quickly and allow them to get an idea of who you are, your values and the type of teacher you are as well as being easily able to find basic information like when/where and how much your classes are.

Take it back to your Ideal Student – what do they need to know? Answer that question on paper, then give them a journey through your website that gives them all those answers.

DIY

Yep, you can do it yourself and you don't even need anything beyond basic computer skills. This is great if you're not familiar with web or user experience design as you don't have to do any of that and you know everything will look and work as it should do. Plus, it is incredibly cost effective to get started.

Platforms like Wix or Squarespace are providers who offer templates as well as custom build options for your website.

Wix is the more affordable option. Wix is perennially popular with many yoga teachers (including me!) plus has lots of additional applications like their free booking system, Wix Bookings, included in the annual subscription price at time of writing. Squarespace is slightly more expensive but is more design led and fancy with a wider range of choice.

Both platforms have ready-designed templates which you can then personalise with your own images, fonts, colours and wording. There are extensive guides and support available on their websites, so if you get stuck or something doesn't work properly you can easily get support and, in some cases, have issues fixed for you.

Another platform you might have heard of is Wordpress. Wordpress can be (in my experience) temperamental and needs an expert pair of hands to code and build your site for you. There are template options available with Wordpress too, and there is a lot of flexibility and choice around the possibilities as it is an infinitely flexible platform with a wide range of plug-in apps for all kinds of features.

If you have had a look at the template site option and still feel like this is going to be super daunting – this is when you might want to consider hiring someone to build and design your site for you before handing it over to you.

If you're really comfortable and have some web design or user experience knowledge, Wix and Squarespace also offer a blank build option to design your own pages from scratch using your own blend of text boxes, buttons, galleries and other drag and drop elements from their extensive libraries.

If you know how to code, you can also use their more advanced options but, personally, I've never found a need to use that – the drag and drop blank build option is more than extensive enough for any yoga business needs.

I'd recommend roughing out the layouts you might want to use on paper first before getting into the building of your pages if this is the route you want to go down.

APPLYING YOUR BRANDING

Earlier on we talked about the foundations of our brand, and now is where we get to apply that work and refine what we've got together so far. Ideally, we develop our branding first and apply it to our website ourselves or using a brand consultant to help us.

Your website should be branded to you! It sounds like a really obvious point, but so often when template sites are used they are not adapted to the specific brand using them and the colours and fonts are left as per the template.

This isn't good because there is a sea of yoga teacher websites out there that are lilac/pink, or earthy toned, with photos of lotus flowers and buddhas all over them called "yoga with [insert name here]" and a person sat in lotus as the logo. It's boring, generic and stereotypical cookie cutter. You're unique, so is your branding. You need and deserve better than this.

As we discussed in Chapter 3, branding is vital. It is literally your outward facing identity and uniqueness, so it needs to be reflective of who you are as well as consistent with your other outward facing marketing, like your Instagram account. You want your Ideal Student to go on your website and instantly connect with your viewpoint and your vibe.

Photography is the first thing that catches the eye on any website and I always recommend organising a professional shoot for your website to make sure it looks consistent with your brand. High quality photography adds professionalism and quality to your site as well as adding an air of authority to your brand. Plus, if what you do looks great...you can charge a great price for it too.

I never recommend the use of stock or generic image banks for websites. Stock/generic images are the images you find on platforms like Unsplash; they're general images designed for brands to use to plug the gap, which is the exact issue – they're generic by design. They aren't specific or unique to you and your brand. You need and deserve better with this too!

If your branding is neutral and calming, you might want to take the pictures indoors in an airy studio space and wear neutral clothes made from natural materials.

If your branding is fun and bright, you might want to shoot somewhere quirky, outdoors or industrial. You might want to wear some bright patterned leggings, unusual jewellery or something you really love.

It's also good to get some more candid and off the cuff images, and some headshot style images so you've got a mix for use throughout your site.

You will also want to consider if you are showcasing asana in your photos. This should always be reflective of what you teach and be aimed squarely at your Ideal Student and not for your own gratification. It is super tempting to showcase showy poses like handstands or poses highlighting a large amount of flexibility, especially after spending a lot of time feeling like you "should" do these poses because you're a yoga teacher (see Chapter 2 for the mindset around this!). The question to ask yourself is: does this pose/photo resonate with who your Ideal Student is? Is it going to appeal, can they see themselves in this image?

If you primarily teach hand balancing then, yes, it would be totally appropriate to showcase lots of handstands on your site and social channels because that would resonate with your Ideal Student. But if you are aiming to teach students who are new to yoga, or even to moving at all, that is likely to put them off and perpetuate the exclusivity issues around yoga too. If your Ideal Student is someone new to yoga or movement, is it better to showcase something simple, like an easy seat on a block with a big smile? Spend some time thinking about the Ideal Student you need the images to appeal to. How do you want them to feel when they look at those pictures? What does this tell them? Grab your journal and jot down a few ideas.

Once you've spent some time reflecting, you can make a list of shots you want to get and provide your photographer with this. If your photographer specialises in branding photography, they might also ask you some questions about your brand and come up with some shot ideas of their own too. It can be a very collaborative and enjoyable experience. Worksheet 5.3 will help you pull a photo brief together.

PHOTO BRIEF

Why is the shoot happening?	E.g. photos for website, marketing materials…
What rights are needed?	
Describe the feel/ look the images should capture:	
Shoot locations	☐ Indoor ☐ Outdoor Add address/maps/what3words reference

Clothing, outfits and props	Outfit 1		Outfit 2	
	Props			

Shot list

Shot	Notes	☑	Shot	Notes	☑

You'll need to consider the colours and fonts you use and where they are applied, and once you've decided make sure these are applied consistently across your site.

A good rule of thumb is 5–7 colours and no more than three fonts deployed as follows:

- a headline colour and font
- emphasis colour – for calls to action like *Book Now*, *Email Me* – two or three colours, one for buttons, one for emphasis boxes and another for subheadings
- body colour and font.

I always recommend that body text should be high contrast (black/navy on white is a good example, if a little corporate) and easy to read. Sans-serif fonts are modern and easy to read without the little "tails" at the ends of each part of the letter.

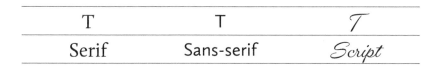

T	T	T
Serif	Sans-serif	Script

It wouldn't be appropriate to use a script-like font for body text – it's too hard to read. However, you might elect to use this for your headings or subheadings.

Once you've decided what you want to do where, it is a good idea to make yourself a Brand Guide using Worksheet 5.4 so you've got a document to refer back to whenever you are creating content, or if you have someone creating on your behalf.

MY BRAND TRACKING SHEET

FOUNDATIONS	
My Why:	
My Aim:	
The How:	
Values:	

Moodboard: Inspirational photos and images to guide your images and creative process

THE VISUALS				
Brand Colour	Colour Name	Hex Code	Swatch	Use
1				
2				
3				
4				
5				

Uses: Background, Accent/Contrast Colour, Call to Action (e.g. Book Here Button), Heading, Subheading, Body Text

THE VISUALS

Fonts	Font Name	Sample (Upper and Lower Case)	Size	Use
1				
2				
3				

Uses: Heading, Subheading, Body Text

EXECUTIONS

Once you're happy with your colours and fonts, set up a few templates in Canva tailored for each of your Ideal Students and types of content. Store examples here or in a folder on your PC.

Making sure it does the job

Your website needs to do a job as well as to look great. That job is to explain about who you are, what you do, how that helps people, how they can buy and how to get in touch with you.

For that to happen your website needs to have sufficient information on it and use clear terms and navigation throughout. It all comes back to your Ideal Student and understanding where they are.

If you had a page called vinyasa classes would they know what that is? Maybe, maybe not. If you put classes instead and then explained what vinyasa is would that do the job? Yes, definitely.

Is the journey clear? If they go and look at classes is it immediately clear how and where they go next to book in or sign up to your membership?

Keep it short, punchy and to the point any time you need to convey information. It is really easy to put loads of words together, but it really doesn't need to be longwinded. Edit and edit again!

Use clear calls to action – *Book Here*, *Email Here*, *Buy* and so on in a specific colour and font. Repeat them throughout the page at key points.

The extras

A contact page is also absolutely essential. This can be a form on a page which visitors fill in and gets emailed to you, as well as listing your email address somewhere on your site.

Blogs are a great way to add your viewpoint to your website and an additional avenue for marketing yourself. When Ideal Students or brands are searching on Google your blog might pop up and they can stumble across you this way. Blogs are also great for getting extra love on Google because the longer people spend on your site reading, the more interesting and valuable it is. Therefore Google shoots you up the ranking, so even more people see your site.

Many website platforms have a linked in blogging platform which you can add straight to your site, ready for any visitors to dive into. Plus, your blogs are ideal things to share in your brand new newsletter! You can also link these to Members Areas in some cases and have specific blogs restricted to your members only as an extra perk.

You need to set up a newsletter. A newsletter is a captive audience who are already warmed up, they know about you, like what you do and want to hear more from you! These are your Ideal Students and they are significantly more likely to buy from you. It is worth the energy cultivating this group of people.

Once you've got their data and permission to email them, you've got that direct contact with your own pool of Ideal Students and potential customers and can build a closer relationship as well as removing yourself from the issues of having your audience solely on social media on rented estate.

Popular platforms include MailChimp and Mailerlite. These are drag and drop editors that allow you to send a newsletter whenever you want to and are free for a small audience size and very low cost once you have above a specific number of subscribers.

You can create a small form which you can then embed into your website footer and direct students to sign up there. You can also link to that form in your link in bio on Instagram or share it on other social media platforms you use, or create a QR code on your business cards or any flyers you have printed.

You might also want to consider offering a sign-up bonus to say thank you for signing up. This could be an on demand class, a printable voucher, a discount code or something else of value to the subscriber. On an ongoing basis you might give newsletter subscribers extra bonuses like early access to classes. Your newsletter is in effect a club and you can sell those benefits and amp up the fear of missing out (FOMO) factor by advertising these benefits on your social platforms to encourage people to sign up.

Booking systems, member areas and payment systems

If you are teaching online, you need to invest in a booking and payment system.

There's a real resistance to this for many yoga teachers for the reasons we discussed earlier on and the fact it is an outlay. However, this is such an important part of teaching online (and in person for that matter) and will make it a significantly more enjoyable experience for you and your students too.

There are lots of different options out there at different price points with different levels of capability and functionality. The choice you make is going to be informed by three different things:

- what will work best for your Ideal Student
- what has the essential capability you need for running your business
- budget.

The system you choose needs to be simple, easy to understand and use and have a clear journey from picking your class and how you want to pay all the way to paying for the class.

It needs to be simple and easy to understand for your Ideal Student, not you. This is a mistake I've made myself. I selected a system initially (costing £20 per month) which required students to navigate to a separate tab if they wanted to buy a class pass, then go to the schedule to select their classes. I spent literally *hours* every week fixing bookings that people had made without class passes that they were wondering why they'd paid more for! I thought it was easy and clear (I'd even written instructions and made notes appear in the process) *but no*. It wasn't. I switched to a combination of software plug-ins to manage my bookings, Members Area and membership/payment plans and haven't looked back. Yes, it's more fiddly for me...but remember – it isn't about me or you. It's about what is best for our Ideal Students. And if that's a bit fiddly to set up initially, so be it.

When you're reviewing the options on the market it's important to think about everything you do currently, and what your plans for scaling are down the line. Here are some of the features you might want to consider:

- Individual class bookings – can people pay for one class on its own?
- Class passes/blocks of classes:
    - Is there a way you can offer multiple classes?
    - Do you require people to block book?
    - Can it handle classes in multiple locations?
    - Can it handle online and in-person classes or will you need to set up two classes at the same time to facilitate this?
    - Does this interface well with the rest of the system?
    - Does it show how many classes each person has left?
    - Is there a reminder facility for when passes are due to expire?
- Link creation and sending for live online classes:

- – Does your booking system integrate with your video streaming software?
- – Is it easy for you to send a link to your attendees manually if not?
- Does the system handle memberships and recurring payments as well?
- Can the booking system be integrated into your website? Is it mobile responsive?
- Can you control the timeframe when people can and cannot book and cancel classes?
- Does the system work well for mobile bookings? Is there an app your students could use to book and pay on the go?

By thinking ahead, you can make sure what you purchase has the most longevity possible and set up a system that works well. A system that works well minimises the times students need to get in touch with queries, cuts down your admin time and makes you money without you needing to be there.

The other consideration is how we get paid for the work we do. Some systems allow you to select offline payments so people can pay you via bank transfer/PayPal/cash. For online classes and memberships this just isn't sustainable or practical. It creates an admin hole of chasing people to pay you, removing access for people who haven't paid or not giving them links, then reinstating that access once they've paid, monitoring who has selected which option.

There is also a range of providers to choose from for taking payments from your students and all these have associated costs. Providers usually charge a small percentage plus a flat transaction fee (20–35p) for each card payment that is processed by them. Some are cheaper than others and charge different fees for certain types of cards, or for currency conversions or cards registered in other countries/territories than your own.

Stripe and PayPal are popular options. They're very simple to set up and connect to your website and booking system and the money is paid directly into your bank account with the fee already deducted. It is a small cost of business (around 40p on a £10 transaction with Stripe at time of writing) and can be factored into your pricing structure.

By making it simple for students to book and pay you're actively removing hurdles from the process and you absolutely make more money from each of your students because of this.

It is also important we touch on budget. Some of these systems are, in effect, free (Wix Bookings, Payment Plans and Member Area is included in your yearly Wix Premium subscription) while others, like MindBody, range from £109 to £479 per month. This is a huge range of pricing and well out of reach for independent yoga teachers as well as many smaller studios.

Some of the more affordable systems do the job just as well but require a few smaller plug-ins working together to do what you need them to do. It really is worth spending a bit of time and energy researching and mapping out what you need the system to do and what you would and wouldn't be happy to compromise on.

Some booking systems already come with a Members Area (Wix Bookings requires you to have a Members Area, for example) but some do not have this facility, which means if you are wanting to set up a membership you might need to invest in another system to support this.

Any system you evaluate needs to be done through the eyes of your Ideal Customer. What is blatantly obvious to you won't be to others. Simple things like each person in class needing to use a unique email address, how to purchase class passes or the need to press "pay" can be incredibly hard for some people who find technology intimidating to grasp.

I always recommend setting up a trial account of your shortlisted systems, popping a few test classes and class passes on there, setting it up as cash payment and giving it to a handpicked group of students who are representative of your wider class population. If you don't have students yet, you could see who fits with your Ideal Customer in your friends and family and ask them. I recommend not giving detailed instructions as you want to understand if the system is easy to use and intuitive or not. Ask them to try out all the functions you want to offer, like booking a single class, buying a class pass and cancelling a class and ask them to fill in a short survey afterwards. You could offer them a discount or a class as a thank you for their help. In my experience students really enjoy getting involved with this as it helps them feel you value their thoughts and input highly.

There are lots of different options available for memberships out there at different price points, and the final selection will be informed by what your unique requirements are.

- Are you offering a single flat fee membership or a tiered membership?
  - Some platforms can do this, others can't.
- Will the Members Area app integrate into your website fully? Is it mobile responsive?
  - If you already have a website with a Members Area which is used for booking classes, it would be a better experience for your students if they can use this for your membership offering.
  - There's nothing more frustrating than embedding an external system within your site and it not being usable on mobile.
- Does the Members Area integrate with your booking system?
  - If you want to offer classes as part of your membership, the students need to be able to book themselves in to class seamlessly.
  - If it is a set number of classes, the system needs to know how many classes they've taken.
- Is there an option for a membership plug-in that your website host already has?
- Is there an integrated video hosting or do you need to host your videos somewhere else?

Websites, booking system and membership systems are often developed in tandem because they're all very heavily interlinked, as this chapter shows. You need a range of elements that all work together seamlessly so your students have a great experience and you have software that is reliable, does exactly what you need it to do and allows you to run your business with less active interaction.

Video editing and graphic design software

If you are recording classes for on demand use you are absolutely going to need some video editing software to pull the final video together. Luckily, there are some fantastic free options out there that work really well for creating great looking and sounding yoga videos.

You might wonder why we need to use video editing software for our videos, right? Well, the next chapter will discuss this in more detail, but if you are filming on a camera (not a camcorder) these *all* have a recording limit of 20–30 minutes. There are exceptions to this rule in very high-end price points and video-only devices. The long and short of this is that you'll need to record your content in sections and stitch them together afterwards. This might sound really complex right now but I promise you it is more straightforward than you might think! (More tips on this in Chapter 7 and I'll show you how in Video 3: How to Edit Your Yoga Videos.)

When we edit our videos, we can also reduce background noise, enhance voice audio and alter the colouration of our video so we end up with a great looking and sounding product that we can charge for, which surpasses the low quality content available for free across the internet. Editing software also offers the functionality to add a title card, overlay music, text or graphics on screen and so much more. Small mess ups and background noise can be fixed easily so you can save most mistakes digitally without having to refilm part or all of the content.

The choice of software will depend on what operating system your computer runs on. Mac computers come with iMovie preinstalled, which is a fantastic user-friendly editing software that is my personal software of choice.

If you are on Windows, DaVinci Resolve is a fantastically powerful piece of editing software, with a huge range of capability, so much so it is used by the film industry. DaVinci is a little more complex to learn initially but offers all the same functionality of iMovie.

Both software suites are ideal for yoga videos, and there's a host of tutorials available on the internet via Apple and DaVinci's own websites so you can learn to use them.

Give yourself plenty of time to do a bit of reading and learning when you come to edit your first video. Remember, anytime you are learning a totally new skill that has a learning curve it is best to take as much pressure off yourself as possible so you can experiment. Refer back to the tips in Chapter 7 and Video 3: How to Edit Your Yoga Videos, which can be downloaded from https://library.singingdragon.com/redeem using the voucher code JEWZDYR

The final software I recommend for any yoga teacher is graphic design software. Graphic design software allows us to create visuals for anything and everything: websites, social media, title cards for our membership videos, flyers, business cards and anything else we might need.

Canva is a free web- and app-based platform just for this and it is excellent because you don't need to be super design savvy to use it. There is a free version which limits some features, and a paid Canva Pro version (currently from £8.99 per month on an annual subscription) which is what I would recommend. This gives you full access to Canva's extensive library of graphic elements, lets you save your choice of colours and fonts and also resize existing artwork for new purposes, which dramatically cuts down the amount of time you need to spend when you need new graphics.

Insurance and other legal obligations

For any and all teaching it is really important to make sure you have adequate cover for your business. You need to be covered in case someone you teach injures themselves and tries to sue you for damages.

Not every insurance provider will cover online teaching on a live basis or for on demand content as standard. Some do on an unlimited basis, some have restrictions and policies such as maximum numbers in a class or require you to use a legal disclaimer on every piece of pre-recorded content you create. Some insurers also do not cover you for teaching overseas or in the USA.

If you are a member of an organisation like Yoga Alliance Professionals, these memberships sometimes come with a level of insurance cover as standard.

Carefully check any insurance policies that you have in place to ensure you are covered for what you are planning to do, and if not obtain additional quotations for the extra cover that you need.

If you are a teacher who uses music that is subject to royalties in your classes, you need to ensure you have the appropriate music licence for where you live to allow you to play music for commercial purposes. You also need to ensure that the source of your music allows you to use that platform for commercial use; many do not allow this and can sue you for breach of contract if you use their products in an incorrect way.

If you are selling your classes into the EU or other global markets, you may need to also register for VAT (or the country of origin's version of this taxation) and pay this tax within this country. Make sure you have an accurate record of where your students are based so you can keep a record of what needs to be paid where to who. I recommend that you consult an accountant/financial advisor to help you with this if you are UK based and are selling outside the UK.

Chapter 6

THE EQUIPMENT

There's no way around it: teaching online in any format requires a fair bit of equipment to create a high quality product that people are happy to pay for.

Filming on an old phone without lights or a microphone was something you could possibly get away with in the pre-COVID world, but that certainly isn't the case now. Students expect great video, lighting and audio so they can have a brilliant class experience and teachers everywhere are having to level up their equipment to meet this growing need and capitalise going forward.

In this chapter we're going to talk about the different types of equipment that you can buy and use. Some is multipurpose so you can use it for online live classes as well as on demand content, some is sole purpose.

To ensure this chapter has longevity, most of it is at a broader level rather than going into specific equipment, with the exception of equipment that I think is truly exceptional and worth a mention in its own right (all models correct at time of writing in Spring 2021).

Video 2: The Equipment can be downloaded from https://library.singingdragon.com/redeem using the voucher code JEWZDYR

The hierarchy of importance

1. Sound – most important.
2. Light.
3. Visuals – least important.

I know this might be surprising, but believe me! Sound is the most important aspect of your online teaching toolkit. Why is that?

Think about when you are in an in-person class... you might be upside down in a down dog, folded towards your chest in a forward fold so you can't *actually see* your teacher. You are relying on their dialogue to know what's coming or any options that are being offered (or you take a quick cheeky glance and see what the other students in that space are doing and follow them).

This is exactly the same online. Your students need to be able to hear you clearly in terms of volume and the audio quality and with consistency of volume and quality as you move. If you don't have a mic, or something that isn't well suited to yoga or movement, that will compromise the quality of what you're creating.

I put visuals at the bottom of the order of importance for a couple of reasons. Audio files are also smaller (even high quality ones!) than a picture so you can transmit great audio in your streamed classes even on a bad internet day. Second, HD video is massively data heavy and going too HD in live streamed classes can make the picture drop out on the student's end if they don't have a fast download speed and also create disassociation between the image and the dialogue.

If you are uploading 4K HD classes to your on demand membership they are ginormous files that take hours to create in your video editing software, render out as complete files and even longer to upload. You could quite feasibly spend 8–9 hours trying to create and render a video file before you're even able to upload it to your membership, which isn't a good use of your time. For a yoga class that's being streamed on demand, the ceiling limit is your student's download speed. It's better to go for a balance of size and high quality so students can actually do your class and not have it crashing or pixelating because it's too huge for their internet to cope with.

Light is more important, because no matter how great your camera is...if it isn't getting enough light the picture will look like you've rubbed a thumb across the lens and be grainy. To get the best out of your camera and the sensor inside it, the brighter and higher quality the light is, the better.

It is far more cost effective to spend a smaller amount of money on some great quality lights than spend thousands on a high quality camera you can't get the best out of because the light in your space isn't good enough. The next chapter will give you some tips on setting up all your equipment and how to get the best set up in the space you have.

Sound: microphones, headsets and peripheral equipment

If you are teaching classes live and your microphone is built into your camera device (laptop, phone, tablet, camera) you are going to be too far away from the microphone for your voice to be picked up clearly and consistently as you move around your mat teaching.

Yoga teacher forums across the internet are full of the question, "what mic do I need to buy?" and there isn't one single answer here; this is again led by what you want to do, how you teach and, if you are creating on demand classes, what you are creating those with.

Microphones are expensive pieces of equipment, so it is absolutely imperative to make sure what you buy suits everything you want to create and offer now and in the future. Cheap microphones often don't produce excellent sound and don't offer longevity. It is the one area that I would recommend the majority of your budget goes into as a priority, for the reasons explained in the previous section.

There are so many different kinds of microphone on the market, with their own specific terms and uses. For teaching yoga, we don't necessarily need to dive into the technical level of how these capture sound; we're more interested in the style of wear and how that translates for the application we're interested in.

- Stand microphone – a microphone mounted on a stand, wired, usually which you plug into the camera device you are recording on.
- Lavalier microphone – a microphone you wear on your top. These can be wired to a transmitter which transmits the audio to a receiver plugged into your camera device.
- Headset microphone – a microphone you wear on your head. These can be a standalone headset which you can plug into a separate transmitter/receiver or have a transmitter built into the headset.

Stand microphones are primarily used for lecturing, podcasts and any scenario where the person whose audio is being captured isn't moving around or being recorded on video. In the yoga world this could be someone who records audio yoga nidras or meditations rather than mat-based practices.

Lavalier microphones are best suited to video where the subject is visible as the microphone is small enough to conceal and won't distract attention away from the subject in the video. This could be someone delivering a video workshop or lecturing at a teacher training. You can also use these in the same way as stand microphones if you use a base or adapter.

A headset microphone is best suited to mat-based classes where the teacher is moving around. Headset microphones are positioned very close to the corner of the mouth, so every word is clearly captured, no matter where you are positioned or how you are moving.

If you were wearing a lavalier microphone on your chest, as you move you could brush it or lie on it, introducing feedback into the audio feed that won't be easy to tidy up in editing afterwards. Also, when you twist or backbend, your head is further away from the microphone, so this introduces inconsistencies in the sound level of the audio feed, becoming muffled as you round and sounding distant as you twist away. This is also an issue with using a stand microphone placed next to the mat as you move closer and further away throughout your practice.

Microphones are available wireless and wired. Wired models have limitations as they need to be plugged in so you can use them; wireless models do not. Some wireless models are wireless between the receiver and the transmitter, but the transmitter might have a wired mic to be clipped on to the chest. This is okay if you aren't moving too much, but for a yoga teacher who is constantly moving dynamically if the wire gets a break in it from heavy use the whole unit is rendered unusable.

The other consideration is the devices you are using to stream and/or record your classes on. If you're teaching live classes and creating on demand content, you need a microphone that you can connect to your computer (probably using some peripheral cables, depending on your computer) and to your camera too via the microphone socket. Not every microphone is compatible with a camera, and others won't work with a computer.

A popular choice of many teachers who teach live online classes is Apple Airpods. If you already have them, it's certainly a good way to get started. If you want to use a camera for recording on demand classes, or you don't have an iPhone or Mac, this option isn't going to work for everything you want to do. There are significantly higher quality products out there that work with a wider range of cameras and computers and offer better sound quality at a comparable price. If you are buying from new, I'd recommend choosing something else.

My microphone of choice is the RØDE Wireless GO. This is an absolutely exceptional piece of equipment for any yoga teacher that offers you total reliability, it's so easy to use and works with laptops (Mac and Windows) and cameras with a microphone port too.

The RØDE Wireless GO is a wireless microphone receiver and transmitter. It has a long battery life of around seven hours, so you can use it a few times before you need to charge it and you just need to turn it on to use it, ideal for a busy yoga teacher. This is a hybrid microphone straddling all three categories as it has a microphone built into the transmitter, so you can wear it on your top like a lavalier microphone and it also has a port so you can add a peripheral microphone to it.

I personally recommend a headset mic (without receiver/transmitter), then plugging this into the Wireless GO receiver for mat-based classes, as a lavalier for workshops/lectures on camera and clipping it onto a tripod for any podcasting or audio recording.

You've then got a product that is infinitely flexible without having to invest in duplicate equipment. The only additional investment you may need to make is some cables to connect into your PC, depending on the model and what ports you have available.

Lighting

Lighting is a critical element of any online yoga teacher's kit. It allows you to create a consistent visual experience regardless of the weather conditions or the time of day you are teaching. Great lighting also allows you to get the absolute best out of the camera equipment you are using.

A really common mistake is blowing the budget on a really expensive camera, not investing in lights at all, then being upset at the quality of the video in low light conditions. This could be late afternoon when the light fades, or just trying to film on a cloudy day. It isn't something that is easily fixable digitally, so classes you film affected by this basically end up being a waste of time and totally unusable.

Cameras work by capturing light being reflected off objects in front of it back through the lens and focusing this onto a sensor panel inside the camera which takes this information, processes it and creates the images you see in your video.

A way to understand the importance of lighting is think about being in a pitch black field – you can't see anything, right? There's no light. Your eyes need light to see, just like a camera. If you switched on the flashlight on your phone, you'd be able to see a few feet in front of you but things a little further away would be a bit hazy and you wouldn't be able to make a lot of it out easily. If you changed the phone for a handheld high-powered flashlight, you'd be able to see a lot more of the space around you and in better clarity. Because the light is better quality, brighter and a slightly different tone, you are able to see more.

Your camera is exactly like this. When the light is bright and a clear daylight tone of light, more light is being bounced off the objects (in this case, you on your mat) and is focused into the camera so you end up with better pictures. When you film in lower light conditions not as much light is coming back into the camera, so the clarity of the picture really suffers.

There are lots of different types and styles of lighting that you could choose for lighting your yoga classes. In this section we're going to touch on the main types of lighting we as yoga teachers would be interested in, as all the products on the market are fairly similar, work well and I haven't found a standout product as yet. For teaching we will need continuous lighting. This simply means the light source is always present, instead of a flash gun which turns on when the camera shutter is pressed in static photography.

Ring lights are small LED lights mounted on a tripod. There are a multitude of different sizes of these on the market, some with phone mounts, smaller tripods and larger versions also. Ring lights fall into the category of task lighting. This means they are designed to focus light in on a specific subject that is up close to the light source, like a lamp on your desk. Ring lights are commonly used by beauty bloggers and make-up artists to light the face of their clients so the detail of make-up can be seen closely.

If you are teaching a mat-based dynamic class, a ring light is not going to be a good choice as the light will focus on a specific point rather than lighting all of you evenly. However, if you are teaching an online course, meditation class or something where you are teaching from a seat with the camera very close to you, in a headshot set up, a small ring light would be the perfect choice for this specific way of working.

Softbox lights are collapsible and adjustable lights mounted on a tripod. They usually fit a high-powered halogen or eco-friendly bulb. The light has a reflective coating inside which bounces the light around and a white diffuser panel attaches over the front of the bulb spreading the light around the space. The benefit of this kind of light is that it is soft and long. It lights a large space with a daylight tone and a soft quality that makes your footage look like it's been shot in perfect natural conditions, even if it is the depth of winter and dark outside when you are shooting.

Softboxes are an excellent choice for anyone teaching any classes on a mat where you are a few metres away in a space. They also work well if you're filming something closer up, eliminating the need for duplicate equipment. The fact that they're portable pieces of equipment is really good, especially if you need to travel with your equipment or are filming at home if you don't have a dedicated yoga space.

LED panels are another choice; these are pretty much identical to softbox lights in terms of the principles of how they work and their benefits. The downside is that these are a lot more expensive to purchase, and to replace if there are any issues with the light source. Therefore, for yoga teachers on a budget a softbox lighting kit containing at least two lights will be an excellent affordable choice and provide a huge uplift in quality for the outlay.

Cameras and webcams

The chances are you are going to be using a couple of different camera options for your classes. If you are teaching live online classes, you'll most likely use a webcam. For on demand content, you're going to use a camera to capture that content.

Webcams and live teaching/recorded Zoom classes

As we discussed earlier, having video quality that is too high can be incredibly detrimental to the class experience for your students. If you have an average quality internet connection and are trying to stream 4K ultra HD video from your fancy camera to a large class who are all also transmitting video on the call you might end up with a whole host of issues like the video stuttering or freezing and the call dropping out for you and for the students.

The focus here is finding a balance of decent quality and clarity so we can keep the feed stable by not overwhelming it with data. The video conferencing software you are using will optimise and reduce the quality of the video to maintain the overall quality of the call. Spending money on another webcam when the one on your laptop is good enough is money down the drain that you could use towards some of the other equipment you are going to need.

For this reason, if you are live streaming classes I recommend using a webcam, starting with testing the one built into your computer and, if that isn't good enough, invest in an external one.

The challenge here is that the quality of webcams can vary incredibly. Some external cameras work amazingly, others can't capture movement in a yoga class clearly because they don't have a great frame rate. Frame rate is the number of pictures the camera captures per second – a low frame rate results in video that jumps if you're making fast, dynamic movement. The higher the frame rate, the smoother the video is. Some built in webcams are amazing, others are terrible and have very narrow angles.

You can also find apps to use your phone as an external webcam, which is amazing, but you might find this a challenge depending on how you've set up your other equipment like microphone, power to your laptop and so on.

To establish if what you have is good enough, you're going to need to do a bit of research and testing. I recommend setting your laptop up in position, with lighting, and asking someone to stand on your mat (if you have someone to hand); if not, you could use a chair to fill in for you.

You can then use another device to log into the call and you can assess the quality of the video from the camera. You might want to use a phone, tablet or another laptop or even ask someone you trust to log into the feed as well and let you know what their opinions are about the clarity and quality of the visuals.

I personally teach using my MacBook Pro (2020 model – 720hp HD) and video is excellent during a stream; it is smooth and clear, and I had lots of student feedback backing this up when I upgraded my laptop. I always ensure I use my lighting set up even during the day to get the most performance out of the webcam (as well as giving the camera lens a good clean before I start!).

This gets a bit complex when we start to think about recordings of classes. I would say this is a situation where this quality is okay in some cases, and not in others. If someone books in for your live class and you offer to send a recording to everyone who is booked in or on request and that recording is available for a short period of time (24–48 hours is common) and then no longer available, I would say the quality of a Zoom recording is absolutely fine in most cases where there haven't been any technical issues. However, if you are hoping to cut corners and not have to record separately for a membership/on demand rentals or buy and keep I don't think this is the best way forward.

You want your membership videos clients pay for to be the absolute best quality because they are evergreen content that will continue to make you money on an ongoing basis. Students simply won't pay a monthly fee for a membership if they can access classes that are higher quality on YouTube for free. They'll sign up, decide the quality is rubbish and cancel and you've lost that person you've worked hard to reach. Because of this, it is well worth spending the time separately recording your classes in the absolute best quality you can.

Of course, there is the option to film your classes on your phone and this is definitely an option to get you started. However, this comes with its own pitfalls. If you have an iPhone you'll know there is one port for everything. This is, frankly, an absolute nightmare if you are trying to film a long class that drains your battery to next to nothing as you're using the port to be able to use a microphone. You also need to have oceans of storage space on your phone and know you have it before you start filming. If you don't, it'll cut out at some point and all that precious energy has been expended and you've not got the footage you need to finish the job.

The other problem that is insanely frustrating is being able to get the footage off your phone onto your laptop so you can edit and upload it. This is another mistake I made when I first started filming content myself using my iPhone. I've had many times where I've nearly thrown my Windows laptop out of the window, I've been so annoyed trying to just find the video and drop it on to the computer. What should be a couple of seconds worth of a job can end up being hours of utter frustration and annoyance. It doesn't work well most of the time, and even less frequently if you are an iPhone user and use a Windows PC or an Android user trying to send things to a Mac. It should work. But it doesn't. I know many a yoga teacher who has been in tears trying to get a video they've promised sorted because of this issue.

I can hear you saying "Jade, why don't you edit it on your phone and upload from there?" Well, trying to precisely edit the start and end of a video, fix any mess ups, stitch sections together and do all of this in a space the size of half a centimetre using your fingers then render the finished video so you can upload it to your video hosting platform without your phone accidentally going to sleep... It will make your head explode and it's a total nightmare!

Honestly. Just don't. If there's one thing you learn in this book, I hope it is this! Avoid this option like the plague if you don't want to give up before you've even started and you value your wellbeing.

This is where purchasing a camera comes in – it's an investment that will make your filming life so much easier and more enjoyable. There are several different types, things to be aware of and considerations when you make such a large purchase.

Standalone cameras

There are lots of different options for cameras on the market. This section will run through the types you may want to consider purchasing for your business.

> DSLR: digital single lens reflex. Professional quality camera type with interchangeable lenses. DSLRs offer a lot of control with unlimited ability to change settings and record in HD and are totally flexible. They are however quite bulky and large, expensive, and can be a bit of a challenge to learn how to use.
>
> Mirrorless cameras: no mirror inside, when you look through the viewfinder you see a small screen. Smaller and lighter than DSLR with the same level of features and customisation options, more expensive usually because the tech is newer. Interchangeable lenses are also available.
>
> Bridge camera: As the name suggests a bridge between a full DSLR and a phone or compact camera. Smaller and lighter again compared with DSLR and mirrorless cameras, but they usually have a fixed zoom lens that you can't change for a wider aspect or longer lens. They often have a slightly lower image quality than a mirrorless or DSLR camera, but still very high quality.
>
> Compact camera: Small and easy to use, point and shoot – ideal for total beginners. These don't always have video capability or quality. They have a fixed zoom lens, which you can't swap out.

RECORDING LIMITS

One thing that is slightly frustrating is the recording limits that are incredibly common on cameras. The majority of cameras are restricted to recording 30 minutes at most at a time. This is for European Taxation reasons. Video cameras are taxed at a higher rate and that is defined legally as being able to record at least 30 minutes of video at once. Manufacturers get around this by restricting the length of recordings to sub-30 minutes; 20 or 25 minutes is common on many cameras.

This isn't ideal for yoga teachers who want to record classes in excess of 25 minutes, but is easily dealt with using a little workaround and some post-recording edits. When you plan your classes, plan in poses where the student wouldn't look at the screen and use these poses to hide the cuts between different sections of video. Down dog or child's pose are examples of great poses to use for this. More tips and tricks for working with recording limits are in the next chapter.

Choosing a camera

The great news here is there is no need to spend an absolute fortune on a camera. If we are recording classes, we need a good quality camera, but we certainly don't need to be going for something top of the range that costs thousands. Top of the range cameras come with a lot of additional features that we simply don't need for recording a yoga class, so there's no point paying for these features!

You might even have a camera in the back of a drawer somewhere that would work for filming your classes on. Personally, that is exactly what I use. I happened to have an old camera lurking around, it's a 16MP Samsung compact camera with a fixed zoom lens and a microphone socket and it records in high definition. The quality is more than good enough, and it meant I didn't need to invest straight away even though it's quite an old piece of equipment.

Think about the size of the space you are going to use as your film-ing base. If you are in a smaller space, you will need a wider angle lens because the camera will be positioned closer to you. In this case, picking a camera that has changeable lenses like a DSLR would be excellent. You can then opt for a wide angle lens so you can capture the space effectively. If you're in a slightly longer than wide space, you might not need to go for a camera with an interchangeable lens as you might be able to find a compact camera that has a lens that is wide enough. It's worth looking at the specifications of some cameras and finding a couple of options.

You will be filming wearing a microphone, so it is important to check that the camera has an input for a microphone and ideally somewhere to mount the receiver for the mic. If you opt for the RØDE microphone I recommended earlier, you can use the clip to attach it to the camera strap or somewhere else to hand, yet another reason why I think this microphone is the absolute nuts.

What batteries does the camera use? Some cameras have internal batteries whilst others accept traditional disposable batteries. It's also worth understanding the battery life of the camera and deciding if you need to purchase more than one battery if you are filming longer form practices or workshops.

A newer feature that is particularly handy is a flip out screen. This means you're able to easily check if you are fully in the frame before you hit record and without having to go back and forwards from the camera checking and rechecking your set up. It can be particularly time consuming to get everything set up, so a handy little feature like this saves quite a lot of time.

What does the camera record on to and how does that link with the laptop you use? Many cameras record onto SD cards, some also have internal storage. When you've finished recording, you'll need to be able to get the footage off your camera and onto your laptop. As we touched on earlier, this can be way more convoluted than it needs to be. Can you connect via a cable or use a SD card reader? If you are using an SD card, do you need to format it first so your computer can read it? If you are a Mac user, you'll most likely need to do this first before you start filming. All details that are really small but incredibly frustrating if your laptop won't read your SD card and you can't get to your footage.

The peripherals – the little bits and pieces to make life easy
It's also worth covering all the smaller bits of equipment because they do make all the difference, either by making it easier for you to get your work done, or by improving the quality of what you film.

TRIPOD
I would always say a tripod is worth investing a little bit of budget into as it lets you get the best out of your other expensive equipment. The higher end models aren't necessary but something mid-range sub-£100 will do the job and make your life a million per cent easier.

It's really tempting to use a ton of yoga blocks to balance your laptop or camera on, or wedge your camera in a shoe (we've all done it!). Problem is, it's a tricky set up to get right every single time, requires lots of trial and error and lacks consistency each time you film.

Never underestimate the importance of a great sturdy tripod. If you teach on a suspended floor at first floor level or in an older property and you're jumping about or flowing around your tripod can move slightly as you send vibrations from your movement through the floor, then the camera can move and this affects the quality of the footage you are capturing.

It's important to refer to the camera you are using and check on what mounting system it uses – most have a little threaded hole on the bottom for a tripod mount. The tripod's mount has a threaded screw on it which you screw into the bottom of the camera for a firm connection with the tripod, and sometimes a pin too. This mounting plate is often removable from the tripod for quick and easy docking with the camera.

It is also worth seeing if you can source a tripod with a hook on the bottom so you can hang some weights off the bottom of the tripod to secure it. You can buy specific weights for this or you can go for a more DIY approach (a big paint can full of stones is my solution – I mean, why spend a chunk of money on a sandbag?!). This is particularly handy for those teaching on a suspended floor as it offers an extra countermeasure against vibration, or if you're teaching outside you aren't risking your expensive camera getting blown over by the wind and damaged.

A tripod should be sturdy with solid feet, chunky legs and a lot of adjustability so you can tailor the height and all the different angles and lock them into place, so the camera doesn't droop or move whilst you are in the middle of filming or when you need to stop and start recording again. The cheaper entry level models on the market have thinner legs, less adjustability in terms of height and angles and don't have the handy features like the hook.

SD CARDS

Get a couple of SD cards. I recommend one that you use when you're filming your class, then your second one is available for use the next time so you can alternate the two between each class you film.

Always format your SD card to your laptop *before you film anything* for the first time. This is the most frustrating problem in the world. You pop a new card into your camera, spend hours filming and teaching some amazing classes, you go to transfer the footage on to the computer and the flippin' thing won't read. It's gut wrenching. Sometimes you get lucky, and the computer will decide to format the card without losing the footage. Other times, it's gone and been wiped. So, always (especially if you use a Mac) dock your SD card straight out of the packaging, format it and then get on with your filming.

Lots of teachers prefer to film all their content, then edit, render and upload multiple classes at once ("batching" tasks together), while others create on a class-by-class basis. Both ways of working are totally valid.

If you're filming a large volume of content at once, you may find that your SD card fills up incredibly quickly, so this is where an additional one is handy as you won't need to delete anything before you are ready. If anything goes wrong and you've been switching between cards during a filming day, if there has been an issue with one of the cards, at least you haven't got to refilm absolutely everything.

SD cards aren't immune to technology fails. Sometimes they decide they don't want to read or need reformatting and you've always got a fall-back card to use without having to dash out to your local tech shop and fork out loads of cash for the convenience of getting another one the same day.

BATTERIES

If you're someone who likes the batching approach, you may want to consider investing in an additional battery for your camera so you can swap and carry on filming the rest of your content with minimal interruption.

If your camera uses generic batteries, it is well worth investing in a couple of sets of rechargeable batteries. It's so much cheaper to run your camera in the long run, and it's super easy to have one set charging whilst the other set is in use in your camera.

EXTENSION LEADS

A lot of softbox lights have quite short power cords, which might be limiting if you don't have a lot of power outlets within your space or if they're not quite in the right place for your ideal set up.

Purchasing an extension lead for each of your lights is a good investment and an easy way to increase your options for plugging all your gear in and flexing your set up to suit.

EXTERNAL HARD DRIVE

You're going to need somewhere to back your classes up to, and your raw footage if you're batching your content. Video files are so huge, an external hard drive is the best bet to allow you to store everything you need without clogging up your laptop.

These are incredibly affordable now and you can get around 1TB of storage for £50. This is plenty to start with, and you can always buy additional ones as and when you need them, rather than forking out a large amount upfront for one with a huge capacity.

When you're researching, check if the drive is compatible with the operating system of your laptop. External hard drives for Mac are a little more expensive; some Windows ones do work but require additional software plug-ins to allow the Mac to read and write to the drive.

CASES

Grab yourself a couple of tech cases – one for your camera (especially if you are using a larger camera like a bridge or DSLR) and one for your mic, cables, connectors and all those bits and pieces.

This keeps all your gear together so you've got everything to hand for the job. If you are travelling to film at another location it's really helpful and stops you from leaving anything crucial at home and also protects your precious equipment from damage.

Chapter 7

TEACHING TIPS

*Getting the Best Out of Your Equipment and
Tips to Make Your Online Space Great*

This is where we're going to talk about how to set all your equipment up as well as some little tips and tricks I've picked up along the way to enhance the in-class experience for your students and to make your life easier as a teacher.

As always, there'll be suggestions here on where you might have some variation depending on your specific teaching style and some recommendations for set ups that work well from my own research and development.

Your teaching position: an overview

How you set up where you teach from is the fiddliest part of getting yourself online. There are so many different things to consider, and it'll all depend on the space you have available and how it is laid out. Trial and error is the name of the game here, as well as giving yourself plenty of time to reflect on the options you are exploring.

Establish the options: where you are in the space

Spend some time experimenting with set ups when you aren't under any pressure or obligation to be ready to teach in a few minutes. The most immediately obvious option isn't always the best one or might throw up unexpected issues, so don't be afraid to really take your time over this.

The space you are teaching in needs to be clear of obstructions and with a good amount of distance from furniture that you could hit your hands or feet on. It might mean you need to totally rearrange the space each time you teach or film and allow time to do this.

Once you've moved any furniture in the space out of the way, you may find that there is more than once position you could have your mat in that allows you to be in camera shot. You want your mat positioned far enough away that the entirety of your body is visible when you're stood up with arms over head and clearly visible when you're down at floor level too. Many teachers also like to use circular or crossed mats so they are able to teach face on, so it is also worth checking on the viability of this option in the space.

Grab your camera/s. If you are streaming live classes and pre-recording on demand content, you may find your set up for each style of class is different based on the lens of your camera and how wide or narrow the angle is.

A good rule of thumb is that the camera should be aimed at you somewhere between hip and chest height, and in line with the centre of your mat. You might need to be creative if you're using a laptop and use blocks, chairs, tables or whatever you have to hand to sit your laptop on to. You can also play with tilting the lid as well as how far away from you the laptop is. Start initially with your camera about 2.5m away from you – about the length of 1.5 yoga mats as a rough point, then adjust from there. If you teach meditation or floor-based classes, you can certainly explore the camera being closer and lower down specifically for those classes.

For live streamed classes, you want to be able to see your computer screen clearly without obstruction. If you have students who leave their cameras on, you can see what they're doing providing you the opportunity to offer them valuable feedback and adjustments verbally as well as know they are with you. Another option is to plug in an external monitor to your laptop and display your screen on this, positioning it out of shot but somewhere you can see them in a bit more detail. Of course, this is all a bit dependent on how people have their laptops positioned. Guaranteed it won't be as well positioned as yours, so you'll probably be able to see belly buttons to knees and not a whole lot else, but you'll have a rough idea at least and be able to add value the experience for your students.

Light: natural and artificial
Any windows ideally need to be behind the camera or situated off to one side of the room, but this isn't always possible depending on the layout of your space. It's important to avoid shooting with a window behind you as this can create issues with the light consistency and quality, leading to

an "eclipse"-like effect where you appear in silhouette rather than being clearly visible.

Space will also be needed for your lighting to be positioned out of shot and connected to power, and for filming on demand content space for the camera and tripod where you can easily get to it and for streamed classes where you can see your students on screen easily too.

I'd recommend using a pair of lights for the most flexibility. Each light should be positioned high, and slightly angled down towards your mat, one on each side of your camera in roughly the same position. This ensures you are lit evenly from both sides and prevents shadows being cast across your body onto the wall behind you. If there isn't space for two lights, one light positioned directly behind the camera is another alternative. You can also opt to add a third light behind your camera if you have lots of space, but the results with two are more than good enough.

If it is a night-time class and dark or a dull day you may also want to review any overhead lighting options in your space. It can sometimes be really helpful especially if you have spotlights to add a little more light in a slightly different tone. If you have more ornamental lighting in your space it can get in the way if you're a taller person or be distracting if it is clearly in shot.

Spaces that are painted a very bright white can also create challenges, especially if the wall you film against is next to a window that has a lot of sun on it throughout the day. White is a reflective surface, and the wall reflects the light from your lighting and the sun back into the camera. This can sometimes cause issues, the camera's light sensor can struggle focusing and refocusing as you move, depending on the sensor in your specific camera. This creates footage where the camera is very clearly struggling to focus and refocus on you, which is distracting for anyone watching the footage and it isn't something that can be fixed in editing.

If this is something that happens to you it is worth considering decorating or adding to the wall you film against to break up the light being bounced around or adding some lightweight window coverings to diffuse the natural light coming into the space.

The look and feel of the space
It's also ideal if the space isn't too visually busy. Sometimes lots of pictures, personal items, furniture and so on are distracting and not the most professional set up for an online studio space.

However, you might choose to have a uniquely identifiable look and feel to your space that is in keeping with your brand. My own studio space has a distinctive wallpaper in keeping with my branding on one wall only, which serves as the backdrop I teach against, which is appropriate and appeals to my Ideal Student.

This also serves as a way of managing the "light bounce" issue I mentioned earlier and dulls down any reflections from the wall back into the camera's light sensor, meaning I get great quality footage, no matter how bright the space is or the light quality variation day to day or throughout the year.

Summary

This is an area for you to use your own judgment on what you feel is and isn't appropriate and what fits with your brand or not. If you're not sure, it is well worth filming a few short test sequences on different days and times, and watching them back to see what you think and sending this footage to a few Ideal Students in return for some feedback on the quality and clarity of the visuals.

Criteria for a great teaching position:

- mat positioned in the centre of the frame of the camera/laptop
- lights positioned at each side of the camera, pointing slightly down towards the mat
- screen positioned so you can see your class if you're teaching live – make sure you can see everyone in your class. You can use your laptop screen or opt to add an extra screen into your set up closer to your mat.

Music or no music?

Some teachers love to play music in their classes, others don't. When students come along to your in-person classes, you might say on your website that you play music, so they are aware and are opting in to that by coming along.

The boundary is a little bit different with an online space, as you are effectively being invited into their space, and they are being invited into yours too. It's a lot more intimate than being in a neutral space like a studio or community venue.

I'm not going to lie – playing music online for a class is an absolute faff. Sometimes it works, others it doesn't; it can require even more equipment like mixers to make it work properly, which can be a lot of additional cost. The critical thing is getting the sound levels right between your microphone audio and the background music. Too loud and your students won't hear your dialogue. Too quiet and there's no point having it there at all.

A little reminder that you still require the relevant music licence if you are going to play music in your yoga classes that is subject to royalties. Another thing you may not know is that Spotify doesn't allow for commercial use, so even if you have a music licence and then share your personal playlists for a commercial use (like a yoga class) you are in breach of that agreement and can get in hefty legal trouble.

If you still want to go ahead and share music in your classes from your end via Zoom you'd need to play the music from your computer (rather than having the music playing in your space), then share screen and play music/audio from your PC only. You would then need to manually adjust the music volume, so you are easy to hear and the music doesn't take over.

I think the better option is to provide choice on what people want in their own space. I have a series of playlists created and I share these with students when I share the links to class, and a list of props. I also explicitly say they don't have to have music, or they're more than welcome to use their own too. This has the benefit of limiting potential for technical hiccups, meaning I can purely focus on teaching the class well, and lets everyone exercise agency in relation to their yoga experience on any given day.

Power, charging and settings

Really simple: make sure your equipment has plenty of charge in it before you need it and it's all turned on and connected correctly!

There is nothing worse than setting time aside to film or having a class that you need to teach and your batteries being flat. At best, it's inconvenient and annoying, at worst it's unprofessional and can really affect the class you're about to deliver.

If you're filming on demand content, I recommend charging your camera and batteries the day before and mounting your camera on your tripod, so you are ready to go. If you're streaming a class, check your microphone battery levels a couple of hours before so there's plenty of time to plug them in if they need charging. Some have larger batteries so will last multiple classes, others don't so it's important you check every time.

I'd also recommend 10–15 minutes before you start recording or teaching to do an equipment check – checking the sound settings on your laptop, checking you're in shot, checking the mic is recording properly (and switched on!) for on demand content. Do a test shot, say a few words, then watch that shot back. It saves you filming a whole wonderful class and then having to do it again because the audio hasn't been captured!

Interruptions and sense of occasion

We all know it is so much easier to get interrupted at home. The doorbell going, getting jumped on by the dog, lack of boundaries and having to find the discipline and will to go to a class when the sofa and Netflix are only a few steps away. It's a super common piece of resistance that students and teachers face all the time.

Interruptions can be as distracting for you as a teacher as for the student. Students dropping out of class and rejoining because their internet connection is bad, or the dog breaking into the room to jump all over you are all things that are going to happen at one point or another.

As is the case with a lot of stuff like this, the key is making interruptions (given their inevitability) part of their practice and making sure students know this is totally okay. At heart, this acceptance of whatever happens is a key part of yoga philosophy and that can even be part of what you teach. One example idea for this might be asking them to observe sounds in other parts of their house – pets, children, the people they live with – and inviting that noise into their practice, letting that become the soundtrack rather than the silence or crafted soundtrack in a carefully controlled studio or class environment.

Putting some boundaries in around practice is another good approach to share with your students. Going to another part of the house, closing the door and making some time for them is the key thing to highlight. Just because they are practising at home instead of going out doesn't make it any less important or essential. They could also have a conversation with the people they live with and ask them to not disturb for an hour so they can get their practice in. Sometimes you might have a student who says something like "the kids would never let me have that time" or similar, so you might even suggest that they get the whole house to join in as an activity to do together.

It's also key that students reframe that annoyance with lack of boundaries to acceptance and you help them to see online practice as something that is special and an occasion just for them, and that the location or circumstance aren't the most important thing. It's about creating value around the home practice experience and teaching how to create a good experience somewhere else.

You might suggest they set up a space for their practice and keep all their equipment in that space. This could be a simple basket, or a shelf in the corner of their bedroom. Realistically, they don't need oceans of space – a few inches around their mat is more than sufficient. You could also suggest they might want to light a candle, use some room spray, put some comfy or favourite practice clothes on and grab loads of props to use in their savasana to make it super luxurious and amp up the occasion.

Community spirit

Interaction in an online space is always a little more limited and harder to facilitate, in comparison to an in-person class. The little chats that break out between students, the banter during a class, the giggles and post-class chatter are all missing, and it's another common objection and reason that people don't always want to come online.

It's relatively easy to make a couple of changes to facilitate this, though. If you are teaching live online classes, you could open your class 5–10 minutes prior to the start and have a chat with everyone as they arrive, share a couple of stories, ask everyone how they are doing or if there's anything in particular they want to work with (if that is something you usually do in your classes) and also offer the opportunity to hang back at the end of the practice if there are any questions or things students want to talk about.

If you are teaching on demand you might want to consider a members only forum/group. A lot of memberships facilitate this through a private Facebook group for members, however this requires a bit of admin time and resource investment and your ideal client might not actually use social media.

A lot of membership platforms also offer this group/forum facility so you might choose to incorporate this into your site. This would cut your admin time down as people who are paid members would be the only ones with access and it also keeps this space within your own website and platform (improving the amount of time students spend on your site and improving your SEO as a by-product).

Your newsletter is also a great place to foster that community feel. You can share useful information like discounts, articles and blogs you've written and create a dialogue by asking for feedback and offering value and little treats in there too. Plus, you can decide who this goes to and use it as a marketing tool as well as a community building activity.

Cueing and demoing

Teaching online is a totally different skill set to teaching in person, let's be completely open about this. It is significantly easier to be able to go and show someone something they need help with when you're in the same room as them and to see if what you're teaching needs to be broken down further compared to trying to do it through a computer where you can't quite see all the fine detail of what each student is doing.

There's an additional complication with how streaming software flips everything around, it can frankly be flipping confusing to understand what the person on the other end of the stream can see and therefore what and how you demonstrate. On Instagram if you are streaming a class on a forward-facing camera, the image is recorded and transmitted in mirror image. This means as you move your right arm it flips the image and it looks like your left (very confusing for a yoga class!); on Zoom/Google Meet/Teams the image is mirrored to you, but it is totally correct to the students watching the class.

It also depends if you are someone who teaches mirrored classes or doesn't mirror. It can add a whole extra layer of mental gymnastics if you are using a platform that streams a mirrored image rather than non-mirrored one depending on the orientation of each individual student and where their camera is in their space. You might be looking at bodies from the left and right sides, from the front or have no visual reference at all if they have chosen to have their camera off.

People also take their cues in a different way in an online space. In an in-person class you might walk the room and people take their visual cues from the other students in class, so you might demonstrate very small portions of your class for additional clarity and rely more heavily on audible cues. Equally you might cue verbally less and demonstrate more in an in-person format. When students aren't in the space your cueing and demoing needs to be taken to an extra level and both bases need to be covered thoroughly.

Students don't have any visual reference except you. Generally, you'll put yourself as the spotlight video feed or ask your students to pin you to the screen so the other class participants aren't visible. So if you have people in your class who are visual learners you are going to find they might really struggle and feel a bit lost if you don't demo and they solely have to rely on listening. This is less of a problem in an in-person class because visual learners can take cues from other students in the class.

Your cues need to also be less context based and move towards very literal and deliberate cues using the body part–verb method. Context-based cueing is often used in person because there are other references in the space that add colour to what you're asking the student to explore.

For example, if you wanted to teach three-leg down dog, high lunge then Warrior 2, you might say something along the lines of: "from down dog, right leg lifts, bring right foot forwards to top of mat, lift up into high lunge, then roll left heel to the floor, opening into your warrior 2", and guide your class through a sun salutation pose by pose and say, "repeat other side", offering less detailed instruction. In an in-person class you might demonstrate this as well or other people in class would be a visual guide to add context. However, if someone walked in and heard you say "repeat other side" part way through the class, they wouldn't know what that was as they don't have the same contextual understanding of the rest of the class.

Body part–verb is a way to teach that is very clear and direction based, which is much easier to understand and process for many people. Say the body part, describe the movement you want the student to make and the action. An example would be arms up in the air, right leg steps back, on to ball of right foot, bend left knee for a high lunge. This creates a clear action and approach to each movement in a simple way.

People also sometimes feel your attention isn't on them at the same level as an in-person class because you are demoing, especially if they are used to seeing you not demonstrate as much. It's worth factoring this into sequencing and having sections that are familiar to your class or using themes to build over time because then you can stop demoing and cue to the people in the virtual room, adding to their experience by making it interactive and relevant to what you are seeing there and then.

It's also a lot more physically draining for you as a teacher to facilitate online live classes in comparison to an in-person one. It's hot under lights, the mental side of dealing with technology is tiring and you might often need to demonstrate more portions of your class than you would do if you were in an in-person setting. It's also much harder for you to get context on how your students are getting on with the practice so you are looking for smaller gestures and tells in their practice, whereas this is much easier when you're in a room with them.

It's really worth bearing this in mind when you set up your schedule so you are working at a level that is comfortable to maintain that isn't going to burn you out.

Quick tips for filming and streaming

Here are a few other tips I've picked up over the years; these are general ones rather than falling into the specific categories we've run through already in this chapter.

- Put a note on your door asking your post person/delivery drivers to not ring the doorbell and leave parcels outside for you.
- Phone and laptop on silent – those notification sounds are really hard to edit out!
- Shut doors – extra layer of sound insulation and gives anyone (or your pets) a visual deterrent from disturbing you.
- Wear outfits you're comfy in – fussy clothing will distract you and get in the way.
- Don't wear head to toe black – this sucks light rather than reflecting it and doesn't look great on camera.
- Set aside twice the amount of time your filming needs to be, e.g. give yourself two hours to film an hour-long class. When you're under pressure you're more likely to make mistakes.

Chapter 8

LAUNCHING YOUR ONLINE OFFERING

Now we know who our Ideal Student is and how to reach them, what our online offering is and have all the supporting systems, technology and equipment in place it is time to take it to market.

There's no two ways about it, launching requires a solid strategy and message as well as lots of time and energy. It can be draining; it can also bring up a lot of emotional and mindset things too.

All launches need three key ingredients: we want to build excitement within our community so they see the value and sign up, high energy to build and keep excitement throughout the process and a super consistent message that is repeated time and time again throughout the whole launch period.

Video 5: An Introduction to Launching can be downloaded from https://library.singingdragon.com/redeem using the voucher code JEWZDYR

What is a launch strategy?

Simply, it is a plan of action that you put into place and execute in a given order. It's often thought that strategy is complex or has a load of science behind it, but it's essentially a fancy word for a plan. That's it!

A launch plan's purpose is to help you get your stuff together and make sure you execute the launch successfully and give it the best shot at success. It shouldn't ever feel like a bind or like you have resistance to it.

It is YOUR launch, so do it in a way that makes you feel comfortable. If you are comfortable, happy and find your own way of selling that feels authentic you're much more likely to succeed and get the best results possible.

Remember, you are a business and businesses exist to serve a customer and solve a problem they have in exchange for money.

Selling and promoting yourself isn't sleazy, gang!

What are we trying to do during a launch?

During any launch we are looking to find our Ideal Students or connect with the Ideal Students in our existing audience and develop what is known as the know-like-trust factor in order to take them along the journey to purchase.

Knowing or awareness is the act of the Ideal Student being aware we exist, what we do and also them quite literally getting to know us. This comes from authentic sharing of content about what you do, the offering you're launching and them having a relationship with you by commenting, sharing, having a chat and all that lovely stuff.

This then fosters that like factor. People ultimately buy from people and liking someone and enjoying what they put out holds a lot of sway. Likeability and being yourself in everything you do is wonderful; people come to your classes because of it so don't be afraid to be you.

Trust is literally that – the Ideal Student trusts what you're saying, sees value in what you are offering and what you are putting out in the world. This can be them getting results from the free bits you pop out on social media, sharing social proof like testimonials or you being authentic about what you do and challenges you face.

Once we've got all of this, selling becomes natural. Your content, relationship and likeability really do the job for you and your job is sign-posting who the offering is for and what each Ideal Student will get out of the offering. Then you'll find people want to sign up because they know your offering will help them.

It sounds a bit like black magic, I appreciate that. Actually, it comes back to it not being about you – everything you do during and throughout the launch is tailored squarely towards that Ideal Student and what they are looking for.

Before we dive into the process fully, let's look at the basic elements in every launch.

The basics: phases and timings of a launch

There are three phases of all launches: pre-launch, during launch and post-launch.

Your timeframe of your launch is for you to decide based on what works for you in terms of sustaining energy and focus on the launch and what your offering is. The during phase of your launch could be short and sharp, which is ideal for lower price point offerings like workshops or special classes (two weeks is a good timeframe for something like this, three weeks if you want to do an early bird offer). It could be a longer timeframe which is ideal for products that are higher like annual memberships (a month or longer).

To decide your timeframe, you first need to define your launch date and then any other key dates that fall within your launch. Your launch date needs to be far enough off for you to have the time to plan your launch and then execute the pre and during parts of the launch process.

The other consideration is the amount of work that needs to go into the product you are launching to get it to a position where it is sellable and ready for those Ideal Students to get stuck into.

If you're launching an online membership and you don't have a website, any classes produced or all the back-end tools in place, you're going to need to allow yourself time to do all of that work before you can start your pre-launch. If you try to do all the build and launch at the same time, you won't get the best version of the product or the launch and you'll end up stressed to the hilt. If you're running a workshop that is a longer version of a class you already teach and you have all your systems and plans in place, then you'll be able to turn that around significantly quicker.

Each project is totally different, and it is down to you to undertake an audit of what needs to be done before you can think about getting into your launch. You can use Worksheet 8.1 to help you with this and confirm you are ready to move into your launch phase.

PRE-LAUNCH AUDIT

Proposed launch date:	Weeks away:	
	Full launch duration:	
Outstanding tasks to complete before launch starts e.g. build workshop web page		☑
Pre-launch date:		
Is this possible?	☐ Yes ☐ No (revise timeframe)	
Does the timeframe feel right and manageable?	☐ Yes ☐ No (revise timeframe)	

You also need to think about what your offering is and use that to inform what your launch is going to look like and what the time critical elements to bear in mind are:

- "Doors Open": Is this a launch of an ongoing product like a membership so your launch date is the first day it is physically available?
  - Are you launching with a launch day offer, e.g. a reduced cost annual membership that is available for a defined period?
  - Are you launching with sign-up bonuses, e.g. extra content/ access to you for a 1:1 for the first X sign ups?
- A workshop/course: The deadline would be the day of your workshop/course or the latest opportunity to sign up, e.g. on the day/the day before.
  - You might offer an early bird discount – you'd have multiple dates in your launch process to work towards in this case: booking opens, early bird ends, workshop/course starts tomorrow so last chance to sign up.

Once you have this information you can start to add some dates in and around the launch. Personally, I like to start with this final go live date and work backwards from there to today's date. Once you've done this, you can see if there is enough time to fit your full launch in between today and that go live date and adjust your timeframe if necessary.

Pre-launch is the phase before we get to the actual launch which involves warming up your audience. This could take the form of little sneak peeks on your social media channels that can become more generous as the launch gets closer, setting the scene of how the offering has come about, some behind-the-scenes content. The aim here is to build some interest and start to cultivate a pot of warm people who are already aware of what you are doing, helping to build some excitement and interest around the offering.

The launch phase is where we introduce the offering formally. All the key information should be included in the first couple of days of the launch window and we want to be super descriptive and tell people exactly how they can sign up.

An important point is just because it is immediately obvious to us how to sign up and what the information is – as we're the one who has designed the offering – doesn't mean it is to Joe Bloggs on the street. It probably isn't.

Take it from me who has had umpteen messages from people – when, where and how much is this workshop on a post that literally says when, where and how much that workshop is. The clearer and stronger you can be with your calls to action (what you want people to do) "Book Here" "Click Book [Workshop Name] in Bio" the better.

In marketing and PR speak, people need to be aware (or know), then they can consider the offering if it suits their needs, whether they like it and you, if it helps them with a problem and ultimately if they want to purchase or not.

For people to be aware and know about us we need to be consistently banging the drum with the message and sharing about the offering. Basically, you need to talk about it until you are sick to the back teeth of it. *That's the right amount.* People need to see things multiple times to take notice and that level of notice and sluggishness around decisions is at an all-time low right now. So, you need to spend even more time banging on about what you are doing than previously.

The other phase here that we cover in launch (and post-launch too) is to collect social proof. Social proof is the little notes people send you in your DMs saying they're excited about it, when people share your posts onto their stories and tag you, the first few testimonials from people who've signed up early. You can then share these as part of your content during the rest of the launch period too, again to build and drive interest around what you're doing all the way through your launch.

The post-launch is always easy to forget about entirely, however it is a great place to sow some seeds for future launches. You can gather yet more evidence and social proof from your Ideal Students after their workshop or once they've had chance to try your membership. You could do this by dropping people a DM or sending them a survey and ask for a little bit of feedback. People are usually happy to do this, especially if they've found value in the offering. You might also want to promote your newsletter to the people who missed out this time around and then leverage your newsletter next time for either early access or extra newsletter subscriber bonuses.

How to go about launching
Your message

As we've established in this chapter so far, the message is essential and key to making sure your offer connects with your Ideal Student. It needs to be consistent throughout the whole of the launch (pre, during and post) and repeated time and time again.

But how do we go about establishing the message? We use all the data and work we've done so far and craft this into a short statement.

We already know *who* the offering is for – it's for your Ideal Student. If you are thinking it's for more than one of your Ideal Customer groups you could look for a common trait between them. An example: if you had female lawyers and male city workers as two of your groups the common trait would be they're both busy professionals.

What problem does the offering solve? Write a short sentence that describes what the offering does. An online membership gives busy professional people the flexibility to practise at any time of day, for example.

What impact does the offering have? This part is about the result of doing the offering and the impact that has on the student. A really good example is professionals who experience severe stress learning relaxation techniques to help them manage their stress better in their day-to-day lives.

We then pull all of this together into a short statement, similar to the one I used at the start of this book:

> The *Online Yoga Teacher's Guide* is here to help you and will cover all the essential knowledge you need to know so you can get teaching online and build a resilient business on your own terms going forward, so even the least tech-savvy teacher can benefit.

Worksheet 8.2 will guide you through this process.

YOUR LAUNCH MESSAGE

What is it?	
Who is it for?	
Where are they now? How do they feel? What is their experience?	
What problem does your offering solve?	
Where will they be after? What is the value?	
My statement	

This statement is the overarching anchor for the different angles you use to communicate with your Ideal Student.

Of course, repeating the exact same words time and time again is going to get boring and it's really hard to maintain the same energy throughout a launch when you feel a bit like a parrot repeating yourself constantly. Using different angles to articulate the overarching message to your Ideal Student is the way forward. Talking about this book I might want to create content that uses the following angles:

- technology: top technology for teaching online
- marketing: launch basics
- membership: different ways to structure a membership
- mindset: how to manage your mindset as a yoga teacher
- confidence: tips to build confidence teaching online.

All of these angles fall out of the wider statement, that is, *the essential knowledge you need to teach online.* They're different angles and ways of talking about that statement as a whole and they all resonate with the Ideal Student (you! ☺).

The main thing is we want to get on the same wavelength and show we hear them, see them and recognise their issues, using their language to explain how our offering will help them on the way to their goals and in their day-to-day lives. Using our busy professionals example, you might want to be really clear, to the point and snappy in your communication – getting to the point quickly in a bish, bash, bosh no-nonsense style is likely to resonate with people who have less time and want to quickly understand *"Is this going to help me or not?"*

Getting the message out there: your content strategy

Once you've got your statement and message and some different angles nailed down, you can start to develop your content plan for your whole launch. The first principle is to understand what the purpose of your content is during a launch.

The content you're sharing is there to take that Ideal Customer across a bridge to purchase. At the start they're on one side, not knowing who you are, what you do, but they're in need of some support – maybe wanting to try yoga but really struggling for time.

They stumble across a piece of content from you, learn something and hit follow – stepping onto the bridge. They see more of your content, walking along that metaphorical bridge, and then you say you're launching a membership (for example) they really connect with you, love your ethos and they go "Oh great! I'll sign up!" That is the job of your content plan during your launch and every other day of the year too. To take people along that journey of awareness, to consideration, to purchase.

All content you produce on social media, your blog, newsletter or anywhere else falls into different streams, or pillars. Your pillars are the themes you talk about across your marketing channels, for example, business tips or yoga tutorials. These pillars are brought to life by the different content types you use, like an image post or a reel. All the content you produce should have a purpose too, whether that is educational (teaching something), community based (helps you build conversations, DMs, comments and shares) or viral (to get more eyes on what you're doing) there's always a reason and a rationale behind every single piece of content. It adds value for the people in your community too, by teaching something, helping them connect, feel seen or bringing a bit of fun.

It sounds blindingly obvious, but social media is just that – social. It's about building that community of people around your business and providing that value and them engaging and buying your offerings because they see the value in everything you do and see how you can help them.

Everyone's process and pillars are totally different, and it always comes back to your community – what resonates with them, who are your Ideal Students and what do they want to see?

In the context of a launch, we want our content to be heavily tailored to support the launch. So, that is going to very much be communicating the message of the launch via our content pillars, using an array of different types of content and different angles.

It is great to have lots of different forms of content going out during your launch covering all the marketing channels you have available to you. That could be Instagram posts (covering single posts, carousel posts, videos), reels, Instagram Video, lives, Facebook lives, posts in local yoga groups on Facebook, blog posts, newsletters, paid promotions on Instagram or Facebook, Google Ads and so much more.

Your content in this period shouldn't be solely sales-led content pushing the offering directly. The content can be educational and add value while providing a bit of a peek at what the viewer will find by signing up to your offering. The idea is for them to think "Wow, this is *such* great information, I've learned something – imagine what I'll get if I sign up?"

As we've touched on time and time again, it is much easier to convert the warm people in your own community first, so focus your time and attention here and skew your content towards these Ideal Students.

The weight of your content during the launch should also lean very heavily towards the offering compared to your usual content. A good figure to work towards is somewhere between 75 and 80 per cent of the content you share in the "during launch" phase tailored towards your offering, and the remainder your usual content. Talking about it once a week isn't nearly enough. Different types of content should be going out daily (if you can) in different places for maximum impact. Remember, you want to be sick to the back teeth of talking about it – that is the right amount.

The remaining 20–25 per cent of your content during your launch should be your usual content tailored towards what you do, sharing your story, proof of how you've helped people and what makes you and your approach different and engaging people as much as possible. All of this supports the launch indirectly because you are helping people get to know you and your business, fostering familiarity, awareness and trust.

There's a way to do it that still feels authentic, good to you without feeling icky about what you're doing. If you aren't comfortable with doing lives on Instagram for example, they do not have to be a part of this particular launch, that is totally fine. You might want to schedule lots of your content in using a scheduling app rather than creating lots of reels and that is okay too. It is your business and your launch. You get to decide what feels right for you to do. These are all suggestions and things that are out there that you may or may not want to consider including.

Here's some examples of the kind of content you might want to include in each phase. The pillar and type of content is entirely up to you as is the execution; these are common points to cover each and every launch.

Phase	Content Considerations
Pre-launch	• Offer sneak previews. • Offering overview – top level details to whet the appetite. • Waitlist – open a waitlist, offer some discounts/extras for people on the waitlist. • Countdown to launch.

cont.

Phase	Content Considerations
During launch	• First day – all the detail. GO BIG! Every detail about how, when, where, why, how much. On every marketing channel you have. • Build excitement – share sign ups, excited messages. • Keep banging the drum – added value content and circle back to message. • Countdowns – discount end dates, booking close days. • Think about momentum – anything to boost and keep it going.
Post-launch	• Testimonials from attendees – add these onto webpage if you're doing a course and open a waitlist for the next round, share on stories. • Announce date of next round/open a waitlist for those who've missed out. • Can you create and launch a passive offering off from the content you have?

Every single piece of content during each phase should have a call to action (or CTA). This is simply a message that signposts people to what you want them to do. Each CTA should be strong, punchy and persuasive. You might elect to change these, particularly in the pre and during phases of launch, because the behaviour you are looking for will naturally be different.

Pre-launch we want to get as many people across the line – first, it means we get off to a flyer and second, we've got hyped people who we can get a little comment from and use that in the during phase of our marketing. Plus, you might want to add an incentive for those who get in on day one of "during".

During we want to go big and bold and super punchy with each CTA. This is the phase where we are actively selling. Wishy washy "oh you can sign up if you want" doesn't cut the mustard here!

Post-launch, you can ask people to drop you a testimonial on a little follow up email asking how they found it with a short survey. It allows you to gather valuable proof as well as further building that relationship and trust factor. Here's some examples of strong CTAs you might want to incorporate in your launch:

Pre-launch	• Sign up to the newsletter. • Register your interest. • Sign up for Early Bird Booking Discount. • Find out more.
During launch	• Book here. • Sign up at link in bio. • Sign up/book now. • DM me. • Share with yoga pals.
Post-launch	• Share your testimonial here.

Pulling your content together

Getting this down on paper (or spreadsheet) is essential so you know exactly what you need to be doing when and where, and what images and copy you need to have ready or still need to create.

Personally, I like to do this on sheets of paper and use Post-it® notes of different colours to map this out. One top tip is to use blank paper for all of the rough work because if you're a creative person (I bet you are as you're a yoga teacher) the lines can rein your creative process and brain in on a subconscious level and stunt your process. This is a tip I picked up many moons ago on my management training, and one I've sworn by since.

Then I transfer a rough version of this to a wall in my office for a few days. This sometimes means I have extra ideas or strokes of inspiration so I add those onto the rough version. I leave the rough version on the wall in view whilst I get this into a digital version on my laptop. Once I've done that, I print out the plan nice and big a week at a time and pop that on my wall. It also means it is super easy to share with anyone who I have outsourced work to and to assign tasks to specific people and track the status of each item and performance.

Add in all your key milestone dates for each phase as a starting point. Once you've got this you'll be able to see all the gaps on paper (literally) and create content for those gaps based on what phase you are in.

Worksheet 8.3 is a content planner template which will help you to plan and track your launch once it's in progress.

Worksheet 8.3

LAUNCH CALENDAR

Notes

Use this template to decide the key dates within your launch.

Start with your go live date first – the date doors open, your first class, the day bookings close for your workshop and so on.

Work backwards from this date starting with your launch phase (period depending on the level of investment and what period of high-energy and attention is sustainable for you).

Add in a pre-launch period to build interest and excitement ahead of your launch.

Monday	Tuesday	Wednesday	Thursday	Friday	Saturday	Sunday

LAUNCHING YOUR ONLINE OFFERING

Reaching out

Once you're in the process of launching you might notice that there are people consistently engaging – whether that's liking posts on Instagram or opening and clicking on links in your emails.

There is absolutely nothing wrong with reaching out to people who you know are engaged by dropping them a DM and saying "Hey, I've seen you've been engaging with the launch a lot – is there anything I can help with or do you have any questions for me?" or something along those lines.

Sometimes people just sit on things for a few days and intend to sign up at the last minute; they might have questions but don't want to bother you; or any number of things or it's slipped their mind. Sometimes that little personal touch – that feeling of being seen, noticed and held as part of a community – can help that person across the line.

At this point it's not your job to hard sell, make them feel obliged into signing up or anything like that. It's not your job to twist their arm and make them feel bad. That is 100 per cent their decision; don't be a dick about it. If they say no, it's not for me this time for any reason – that's cool.

No means no, always. It doesn't mean argue the toss with me. Ever. Always. In every life situation. Respect people's boundaries.

Let them know that's cool, respect the boundary and keep engaging with them. They might be the ideal client next time around and you've done something that has built your relationship, so it isn't ever a wasted endeavour.

The don'ts

Let's face it, nobody likes pushy, dirty sales tactics. There's *nothing worse* than getting a super cold DM from someone trying to sell you utter rubbish. Someone likes a handful of posts, doesn't follow you and then drops you a message saying "Hey girl, I see you're into yoga...buy my MLM Herbal junk". You say no thanks, then they start an argument. It makes me dry heave. Like honestly. It's also not always nice to receive an unsolicited voice note either, it can feel super invasive. There's no integrity or authenticity here, just crappy sales scripts and dated techniques.

Another tactic that falls into the don't category is pushing urgency/scarcity and relying on the fear of missing out throughout the entire launch phase. This can look like "there's one space left" all the way through the whole launch when actually there are plenty, or messages along the lines of "if you want your business to grow you must do this workshop". Again, ick.

It's more than okay to say there are 10/15 spaces on this and keep people updated for information reasons. That comes from a space of helping. One thing that is a particularly popular piece of content in the Instagram world is the Post-it® wall. This involves using some colourful sticky notes (bonus points if they're a brand colour!), and writing the names and handles of people who have signed up to your offering on them and then sharing this list of people on your Stories. This checks the boxes for creating hype about your offering, it's shareable and it also helps people see social proof – other people think it is good and want to join in.

That's very different to creating fear and hanging the entire hat of your launch on something that isn't true. It's not ethical or authentic.

Mindset and launch process

I mentioned right at the start of this chapter that launching is incredibly tough and psychologically challenging. The energy and effort it takes to launch well is relentless; you will find it tiring and you might want to give up.

Impostor syndrome *loves* to rear its horrible head right in the middle of launches because of the nature of how launches work.

I'm going to be straight and say there is always a huge lull in the middle. You will have next to no sign ups in the middle of your launch. That is normal, and nothing to do with you, the viability of the offering or your ability as a yoga teacher.

A typical launch will look something like this graph:

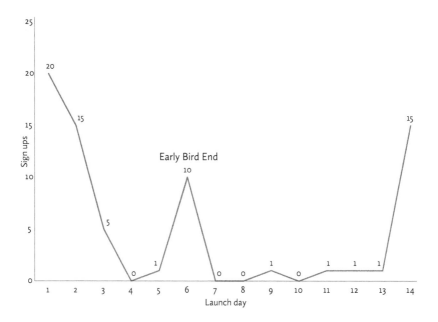

You're most likely to get sign ups right at the start – especially if you've hyped the heck out of it at pre-launch and had a waiting list with some strong early booking incentives like discounts or added value for the first few sign ups.

Then it'll drop off. The incentive for people to sign up immediately is finished, or that's the perception and people's view. They think they won't be in the first few to get that incentive, so they sit on it for a few more days. It absolutely is normal for this to happen and it doesn't mean you're doing a bad job.

You'll get a mini wave part way through especially if you've got an offer finishing. Then it'll go quiet again. On the last day – whether that's the bookings closing, the day of the workshop/event/course launch, you'll get all the last-minute people booking in. It's just how people are.

In experience, you get two types of people – the super organised, want to know what they're doing kind and the so relaxed they're basically horizontal crew. In the middle part of a launch there's not really an incentive for them to sign up or get into action. It's still a week away, the discount has finished, maybe they don't know if they're around yet. So they'll leave it to the last possible second.

Of course, our best frenemy impostor syndrome now wants to pipe up and try to shoot us down. It's screaming things like...

"It's crap – no one will buy this."

"What makes you think you can do this? You're a fraud."

"I'm talking about this too much and boring everyone – they're all going to unfollow."

None of this is true at all. Think all the way back to Chapter 2… It's your subconscious trying to railroad you because, let's face it, launching can be scary. You're putting yourself out there and your subconscious is trying to rein you back in, so you are safe.

Don't listen to your subconscious. It's trying to railroad you.

You've done your research. You know exactly who your Ideal Student is, what their needs are, what transformation they need in their lives. It's fact. Of course it isn't crap, and people will buy it and sign up.

You can do it. A really great thing to do here is keep a little folder on your phone, in a notebook or wherever else, that holds your proof that you do a great job. This can be the texts, emails or DMs people send you saying how much they enjoyed your class, the nice things people say about you. The physical proof that shows you are great at what you do and you are not a fraud at all.

When it comes to the frequency people see you talking about your offering, there's nothing to worry about here either. The odd person might switch off, which is fine, but the people who are there are interested and Ideal Customers. When your offering is designed for them, why would they switch off? If anything, they're going to buy it. It's also important to remember not every person will see every single piece of content you produce; they might only see one piece for every ten things you put out depending on the time of day, whether they are on their phones, if your emails go to their inbox and lots of different factors. When that content has value, they're going to identify with that regardless, even if they aren't intending to sign up. If you are launching a course or programme, even if they don't engage this time, they are certainly warmer because they'll have seen you talking about it and be way more likely to sign up next time. This is why we want to be banging that drum loud and proud, over and over.

It doesn't matter that you know and understand all of this – it's still going to crop up. Especially in your first few launches or the first time you launch something new that you've put loads of effort and energy into.

So how do you deal with this? Make sure you take time out and don't let your launch consume you. It's important to keep an eye on looking after yourself throughout the launch window.

- Make sure you are getting your own yoga practice in.
- Get outside.
- Schedule in downtime!
- Automate as much as you can – schedule posts, email workflows, reminders.
- Make life easy for you – if you're teaching as well can you get easy quick dinners and lunches into the house, get a cleaner or enlist help from your loved ones to do some of the things you usually do? It takes one more thing off your plate.

During the launch phase it can really feel like you are spinning all of the plates managing getting all this content out, tracking performance and doing all your other work as well. It is hard work.

This is where having a robust content plan is going to come into its own. It helps you to see easily what is planned in, what the wording is, the method, what needs to be done when, what has been scheduled already and what the status and who is doing what item is for anything that is outsourced.

Another nice thing to do is add some metrics lines into your content so you can see how it has performed. If you know a particular piece of content has taken a bunch of people across the line to purchase, you can absolutely adapt and evolve the plan during the launch and run that content again in another format. People won't even notice, I promise you.

It's all about launching in a way that feels good for you. Using a plan that is achievable, feels authentic for you and your business that is researched and carried out with lots of energy, value and positivity.

Parting Thoughts

You've made it to the end! Wooooo!

The aim of *The Online Yoga Teacher's Guide* has always been about empowering yoga teachers to take their own slice of the hugely profitable online yoga world and not having to survive on scraps or run ourselves ragged teaching lots of classes.

Online doesn't have to be a big, scary, horrible thing.

It's always been about showing you that it is entirely possible for you to be the master of your own yoga destiny and there's nothing standing in your way. Yes, technology can be a headache: there's new stuff to learn, mindset issues to navigate and lots of other things.

It's all totally doable with a bit of effort, with support, encouragement and an accessible way of explanation and step-by-step processes and systems to support you.

We've worked through all the things you need to know about building your online teaching business from the model you're going to use, the equipment and how you're going to go about getting it out in the world for your Ideal Students to enjoy.

At the start of this book, we kicked off with a short intention setting exercise. Let's circle back to this and examine the journey we've been on together:

Intentions Revisit
Equipment needed: timer, notebook and a pen

- Sit down with your notebook and pen.
- Set a timer for 10–15 minutes.

- Spend a few moments revisiting your answers to our earlier prompts (below for reference):
  - Why did I pick up this book?
  - What are the three things I need help with the most?
  - What questions on teaching online do I need help finding answers for?
  - How do I feel about teaching online right now?
  - How do I want to feel about teaching online after I've completed this book?
- Journal around this second set of prompts:
  - Do I have clarity on the three things I needed help with?
  - Have I found the answers to my teaching online questions?
  - Have my feelings about teaching online changed?
  - How have my feelings shifted?

I bet (and hope!) that your position on teaching online has shifted and our intentions exercise has only highlighted that for you. Sometimes, when the change is right under our nose, it's not always the clearest or easiest thing for us to see.

Before we finish, there are a few final parting business lessons I'd love to leave you with. These don't fit in particularly well anywhere else but they're so valuable it'd be remiss of me not to share these with you.

Social media and the yoga industry

If that yoga teacher makes you feel like shit, less than or like you're not doing a good job – mute or unfollow them. No one needs that in their life! You're on your own journey, running your own business with totally different Ideal Students. So of course, your approach will be different.

You've got your own plan now: you know what you need to do, where and when. Let that give you the knowing that you're on the right path for you.

Other teachers are friends, not foes

You really want to support and uplift other yoga teachers where you can. Being in your yoga teacher community is so valuable, especially if you teach in-person classes too in studios or your own classes. It's where you get the lowdown on issues in the wider community, problem students and any shady studio operations so you can steer clear.

If you're in the UK or the USA, we're lucky to have Yoga Teachers Unions, so again I'd encourage you to get involved and be the change our industry really wants to see. Teaching can also be very solitary as a profession, with odd hours, and it can make you feel lonely as lots of people don't really get what we do. Plus, it gives you a group of people to call on for some support and advice if and when problems show up. Chances are in a group of yoga teachers there will be at least one other person who has experienced something similar and have some wise words for you.

Here are some ideas:

- Refer students to other specialist teachers – like pregnancy teachers if you aren't qualified, for example.
- Invite other teachers to guest spot on your membership and revenue share with them.
- Set up a coffee shop catch up with teachers in your area.

It would also be remiss not to share the things *not* to do. Unfortunately, like any other profession, there is a fair share of idiots in the yoga world. It attracts people with trauma, mindset issues that are deep seated, and often these individuals act from a place of scarcity or lack that can cause headaches for you and your business.

Please don't go out there trying to poach another teacher's clients. It does happen and can look like posting on another teacher's post online, butting into conversations between a potential student and another teacher, putting a banner advertising their classes outside where you host yours or a million other ways.

The adage of "if you wouldn't like it if someone did it to you" is a wonderful test to apply to everything you do. If you research and plan thoroughly, you'll be more than aware of anything that might crop up. Generally acting with good manners and good intentions means you won't fall in to any of these traps.

If another teacher does ever reach out to you because they're not happy with something you've done, hear them out, be gracious, offer an apology and don't do it again – if it's something totally reasonable and you are in the wrong. Basically, don't be a dick and you're all good!

Prioritise your own rest and wellbeing...and practice

When you're in your own business there are always a million things to do, people who need things, classes to plan. As a creative profession, you need to be well rested to deliver your absolute best in each and every class you teach and to develop your business. Schedule your rest and own yoga practice time in your diary and don't compromise on it.

The yoga practice point is particularly pertinent. Our own practice is where a lot of our creative spark and inspiration comes from. So, if we lose our practice, where does that come from? It's tough to teach or plan classes if you're lacking that inspiration and you might feel really stuck and less aligned with your work.

Make sure you make a yoga date with yourself. You could sign up to another teacher's yoga membership online or go to a studio class or an online class. We have so much choice now, the world is really your oyster.

Don't say yes if you want to say no

You have powerful intuition, your gut feeling or inner knowing (whatever you call it). If something isn't immediately a hell yes then it should probably be a fudge no. Saying yes instead of following your intuition can lead you to teaching classes that are paid badly, things that don't align well with your brand or values, that make you feel bad and that drain your energy. As a business owner, learning to say no politely is such a valuable lesson. Here are some lovely examples:

- "Thanks for the opportunity; however, I am unable to take this up at this moment in time."
- "No" – it's a complete sentence. This one is particularly useful if you're being pushed.
- "Thanks for thinking of me, I'm unable to take on additional work right now."
- "Thanks for the offer, it doesn't feel like the right time currently but could we revisit this in the future?"

Sometimes you might feel like you have to justify yourself, but you don't. Depending on the relationship and who is asking, you might want to add some context but it isn't essential.

We're at the end

I hope you're now feeling confident and empowered to get yourself online with a solid plan behind everything you're going to do and that I've shown you that with a bit of time and planning it doesn't have to be scary, and you can go and get business for yourself and work in a way that makes you feel great.

It has been such a genuine pleasure to get to write this book and share this journey with you, and I wish you the best of luck with your new online endeavours.

My inbox is open for you to get in touch with me for any questions or further support. You can email me at jade@prideyoga.co.uk or follow along on Instagram @prideyoga.

Lots of love
Jade x

Acknowledgements

If you'd told me nearly a decade ago when I'd just started my first PR job that I'd eventually write and publish a book, I absolutely wouldn't have believed you and probably said something like "ahhh eff off, no way"!

This book came about because I see day in and day out that so many yoga teachers struggle with business basics and confidence. I was looking for a resource to share, couldn't find anything and started writing and thought more teachers out there would find this useful. So, I did some research, emailed Sarah Hamlin at Singing Dragon and told myself "What's the worst thing that could happen? She might say no. That's not that bad." And that's where this surreal and wonderful project all started!

Huge thank yous all round to Sarah Hamlin, Masooma Malik, Vera Sugar and the whole team at Singing Dragon and Jessica Kingsley Publishers for their belief in this book when I pitched it, their support with questions throughout the writing process and making it the best version of this book you're holding today. Thank you soooo much, I'm eternally grateful for this huge opportunity.

I'd also like to say a massive thank you to my Mum and Dad: Sharon and Martin Wells, my in-laws: Mark and Jac Beckett, Toby Wells, Meg Williams and Baby Wells. You've always been the most supportive and encouraging group; you've read and re-read many drafts of this book over the past few months and been a sounding board for my ideas too. Thank you to all my wonderful friends for always asking how I've been getting on while I've been MIA writing!

I wouldn't have a business without my wonderful yoga students in Oxfordshire either – my Ambrosden crew, Fencott & Murcott crew, the online crew and Pride Pack members. You've put up with my schedule changes, learning to practise online, fewer workshops and my stressing about the writing process over the past few months. I've learned so much from you all; you inspire me daily and I am so appreciative of our yoga community. Thank you for your support.

Thank you to all my yoga teachers, studios I've been to and teacher trainers I've learned from over the years. You've helped shape me into the teacher I am today so I can do something I love deeply every day.

Final thank you goes to my lovely husband, Josh Beckett. You're my biggest cheerleader, you support me to the ends of the earth, and I know you're always there to help me with my dreams and schemes and offer tea and hugs when I get knocked. Now I've printed this for the world to see...can we get another dog please?

Remember, my yoga teacher friend – you can do anything you want to do. No dream in your business is too lofty! Go out there, teach yoga and help as many people as you can.

About the Author

Jade Beckett is an independent yoga teacher, business coach and author. Prior to setting up her yoga business, Pride Yoga, Jade spent over 12 years as an award-winning PR and marketing expert. She now aims to make yoga accessible by making yoga and business easy to understand, helping yoga students and teachers feel confident and find joy in the yoga world.

Jade is based in the countryside outside Oxford, UK, and lives with her husband, two cats and working cocker spaniel. Outside yoga, Jade can be found playing the violin, walking, surfing or trying not to fall off her skateboard.

Endnotes

1 Globally, the online/virtual fitness market was valued at $6046 million in 2019 and is projected to reach $59,231 million by 2027, growing by a compound annual growth rate (CAGR) of 33.1% from 2020 to 2027 (Allied Market Research *Online/Virtual Fitness Report 2021* available at www.allied-marketresearch.com/virtual-online-fitness-market).

2 GlobeNewswire 2020 available at www.globenewswire.com/news-release/2020/12/08/2141452/0/en/Online-Virtual-Fitness-Market-Is-Expected-to-Reach-59-23-Billion-by-2027-Exclusive-Report-by-AMR.html.

3 Caroline Castrillon, "5 ways to go from a scarcity to abundance mindset", 12 July 2020, available at www.forbes.com/sites/carolinecastrillon/2020/07/12/5-ways-to-go-from-a-scarcity-to-abundance-mindset/?sh=374c16ca1197.

4 Wellness Creative Co, "Yoga industry growth, market trends & analysis 2021", 21 January 2021, available at www.wellnesscreatives.com/yoga-industry-trends.

5 Finder.com, "Yoga statistics" (regularly updated), available at www.finder.com/uk/yoga-statistics.

6 Tina Cartwright, Heather Mason, Alan Porter and Karen Pilkington (2019) "Yoga practice in the UK: a crosssectional survey of motivation, health benefits and behaviours", *BMJ Open*, available at https://bmjopen.bmj.com/content/bmjopen/10/1/e031848.full.pdf.

7 Suyin Haynes, "The global gender gap will take an extra 36 years to close after the COVID-19 pandemic, report finds", 30 March 2021, available at https://time.com/5951101/global-gender-gap-135-years.

8 Robert Booth, "UK's first yoga union fights for fairer share of £900m-a-year industry", 4 February 2021, available at www.theguardian.com/lifeandstyle/2021/feb/04/uks-first-yoga-union-fights-for-fairer-share-of-900m-a-year-industry?fbclid=IwAR0X3zsh8URblhXWUG-5bEovhbpUMbfAGcUJHAAS-hSPNxJUzEe_soN1BrLQ.

9 Harvard Medical School, "Understanding the stress response", 6 July 2020, available at www.health.harvard.edu/staying-healthy/understanding-the-stress-response.

Index